DASH DIET COOKBOOK
FOR BEGINNERS 2024

1500 Days of Low-Sodium DASH Diet Weight-Loss Recipes for Managing High Blood Pressure and Hypertension

Includes a 6-Week Workout Plan and a 30-Day Meal Guide for Beginners

JUANITA SCOTT

DISCLAIMER

The information provided in this book is for general informational purposes only. It is not intended to be a substitute for professional medical advice, diagnosis, or treatment. Always seek the advice of your physician or other qualified health provider with any questions you may have regarding a medical condition.

The author and publisher of this book have made every effort to ensure that the information in this book is accurate and up-to-date at the time of publication. However, they make no representations or warranties of any kind, express or implied, about the completeness, accuracy, reliability, suitability, or availability of the information contained within. The author and publisher disclaim any responsibility for any adverse effects or consequences resulting from the use of the information presented in this book.

The dietary recommendations and recipes provided in this book are intended as general guidelines and may not be suitable for everyone. Individual nutritional needs vary, and it is advisable to consult with a qualified healthcare professional or registered dietitian before making significant changes to your diet.

This book may contain references to specific products, services, or third-party websites. These references are provided for informational purposes only and do not constitute an endorsement or recommendation.

JUANITA SCOTT

JUANITASCOTT007@GMAIL.COM

ABOUT THE AUTHOR

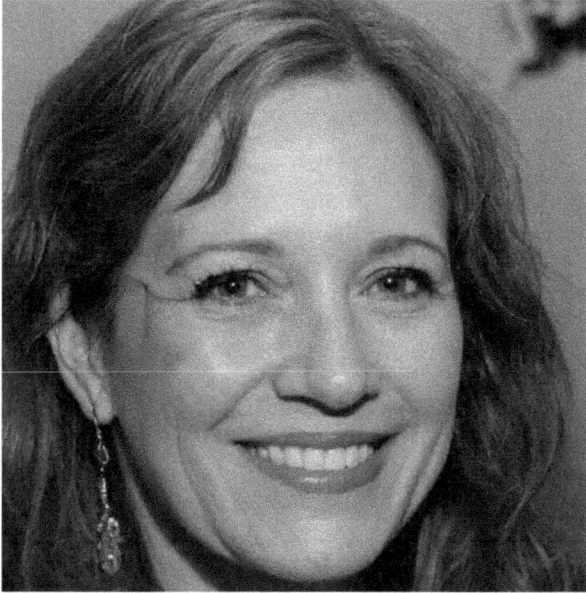

Meet Juanita Scott, a culinary virtuoso, seasoned nutritionist, and dedicated dietitian whose passion for healthy eating and lifestyle has transformed the lives of many. Beyond the artistry of the kitchen, Juanita brings a wealth of expertise, seamlessly blending her culinary mastery with a deep understanding of nutrition to create a holistic approach to well-being.

With years of experience as a chef, Juanita has honed her skills in crafting not only delectable meals but also dishes that prioritize health without compromising on flavor. Her culinary creations are a testament to the belief that nutritious food can be both a source of nourishment and a celebration of taste.

As an accomplished nutritionist and dietitian, Juanita goes beyond the realm of recipes, weaving together the intricate dance of nutrients and their impact on overall health. Her commitment to promoting wellness extends beyond the pages of cookbooks, resonating in every piece of advice she shares with her audience.

Married and blessed with a beautiful family, Juanita understands the importance of fostering a lifestyle that caters to the needs of both adults and children. Her family-friendly approach to healthy living is reflected not only in her recipes but also in the way she encourages households to embrace wellness as a shared journey.

Juanita's unique perspective on the symbiosis of culinary art and nutritional science makes her a sought-after authority in the realm of healthy living. Her work has inspired countless individuals to reevaluate their relationship with food, transforming meals into moments of nourishment, joy, and familial connection.

When she's not in the kitchen or counseling clients, Juanita revels in the simple pleasures of family life. Her dedication to her own family's health echoes in the heartfelt advice and delicious recipes she shares with readers.

Join Juanita Scott on a journey to a revitalized, healthier you. Through her books, consultations, and culinary creations, she invites you to savor the richness of life and health, one mindful bite at a time.

TABLE OF CONTENTS

THE
ANTI-INFLAMMATORY
EATING COOKBOOK

Get Your Bonus Now!!!

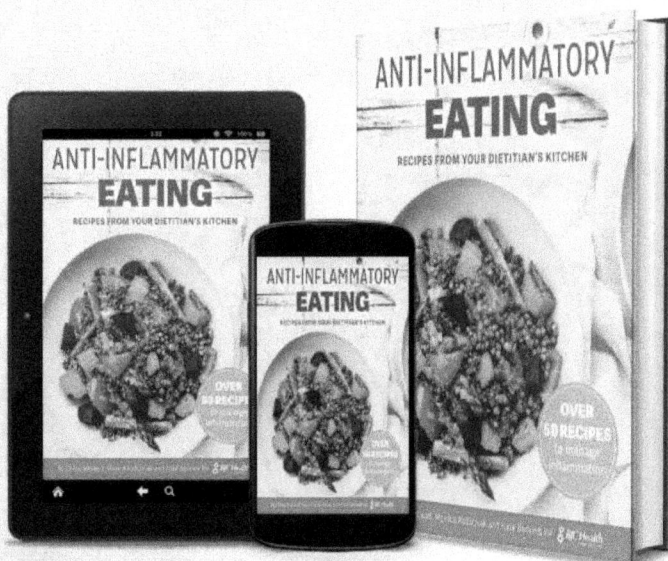

INTRODUCTION

In the quiet halls of my nutrition practice, I encountered a remarkable story that became the catalyst for this book—the tale of Mrs. Thompson, an energetic woman with a heart as robust as her laughter. Mrs. Thompson had walked into my office one day with a glow that defied her age, but her health journey had not always been so luminous.

A few years prior, Mrs. Thompson found herself at a crossroads. Struggling with hypertension, she faced the daunting reality of medication adjustments and lifestyle modifications. A sense of fatigue replaced the bustling energy that once defined her life, and the joy she derived from culinary delights seemed to dwindle alongside her well-being.

Enter the DASH Diet—a transformative approach to nutrition that captured Mrs. Thompson's attention and became the cornerstone of her health revival. As she embarked on this culinary adventure, the changes were not merely physical; they resonated through every aspect of her life.

And so, dear reader, this cookbook is born from stories like Mrs. Thompson's—a testament to the profound impact the DASH Diet can have on one's well-being. As an experienced nutritionist and advocate for mindful eating, I am honored to guide you through the tantalizing realms of flavor and nutrition that the DASH Diet offers.

In these pages, you will discover more than just recipes; you will embark on a journey of understanding. The DASH Diet, short for Dietary Approaches to Stop Hypertension, is not a fleeting trend but a sustainable approach to eating that has withstood the test of time. It is rooted in evidence-based principles that extend beyond lowering blood pressure, and embracing the broader concept of holistic well-being.

What sets the DASH Diet apart is its focus on balance. It is not about deprivation but rather the artful integration of nutrient-rich foods that tantalize the taste buds while nurturing the body. You will uncover the beauty of lean proteins, vibrant vegetables, whole grains, and heart-healthy fats dancing together in culinary harmony.

I know that navigating the world of nutrition can be overwhelming, especially for those new to the DASH Diet. Fear not, for this cookbook is your compass, guiding you through every step of your transformative journey. From understanding the DASH diet to practical tips on grocery shopping and essential tips on how to read labels, we lay the foundation for your success.

But health is not solely confined to what rests on our plates. In a special chapter, we explore the synergy between the DASH Diet and physical activity. Just as Mrs. Thompson discovered, a balanced exercise routine complements the nourishment provided by these recipes. You will find workouts tailored to different fitness levels and a training schedule that seamlessly integrates with the DASH lifestyle.

As we embark on this culinary and wellness voyage together, remember that each recipe is more than a list of ingredients—it is a celebration of health, a dance of flavors, and a commitment to your well-being. The DASH Diet Cookbook for Beginners 2024 is more than a collection of recipes; it is a testament to the transformative power of mindful eating.

So, dear reader, fasten your apron, sharpen your knives, and let's embark on a journey where health and flavor coalesce. May the stories within these pages inspire your own tale of well-being and resilience. Welcome to a world where nourishing your body elevates your life—one delicious recipe at a time.

OVERVIEW OF THE DASH DIET

The DASH Diet, which stands for Food Approaches to Stop Hypertension, is more than just a food plan; it is a lifestyle based on scientific principles that promotes heart health, manages blood pressure, and fosters general well-being. The DASH Diet, created by the National Heart, Lung, and Blood Institute (NHLBI), has received widespread praise for its effectiveness in lowering hypertension and its holistic approach to nutrition.

High blood pressure and LDL cholesterol levels are two significant risk factors for heart disease and stroke. Foods on the DASH diet are high in potassium, calcium, and magnesium. The DASH diet emphasizes vegetables, fruits, and whole grains. It contains fat-free or low-fat dairy products, fish, chicken, beans, and nuts.

The diet limits foods high in salt, often known as sodium. It also restricts the amount of added sugar and saturated fat in foods like fatty meats and full-fat dairy products.

KEY PRINCIPLES

Let's look at the essential components of the DASH eating plan that make it beneficial for treating hypertension and boosting general health. By adhering to these guidelines, you can make positive changes to your eating habits and enhance your health.

1. Emphasize fruits and vegetables:

Fruits and vegetables are a key component of the DASH diet. In fact, it is recommended that you consume at least 4-5 servings daily. The reason for the emphasis on these foods is because they are effective at lowering high blood pressure. One study found that persons with high blood pressure who ate more fruits and vegetables had lower systolic and diastolic blood pressure.

2. Whole grains for heart-healthy eating:

Whole grains are another key part of the DASH diet. They are beneficial to maintaining normal blood pressure because they contain potassium, which lowers blood pressure. Furthermore, consuming whole grains helps enhance blood cholesterol levels and reduce your risk of stroke and obesity.

Incorporating whole-grain options into your meals, such as bread, whole-grain pasta, brown rice, and oatmeal, is an excellent way to establish a heart-healthy eating habit and prioritize your cardiovascular health.

3. Lean proteins for optimum health:

Including lean protein in your diet is beneficial not only for the DASH diet but also for overall health. Poultry and fish are high in lean protein and include critical vitamins and minerals. In contrast, legumes supply both dietary fiber and plant-based protein.

Low-fat or fat-free dairy products, such as yogurt and skim milk, include protein and calcium, which promote bone strength. Incorporating these lean protein items into your meals not only promotes muscle growth but also increases satiety, which adds to a balanced and nutritious diet.

4. Healthy fats for cardiovascular health:

When it comes to dietary fats, it's critical to know which ones to avoid and which are actually good for your heart.

As a general rule, avoid foods high in saturated fat, such as fatty meats, full-fat dairy products, tropical oils, and the like, because saturated fat can elevate "bad" LDL cholesterol and increase the risk of heart disease and stroke.

At the same time, incorporating healthy fats into your diet can help lower cholesterol, normalize cardiac rhythm, and manage high blood pressure. Nuts like almonds, walnuts, and pistachios are excellent sources of healthful fats, as are olive oil and avocados.

5. Lowering salt consumption:

The DASH diet emphasizes reducing salt intake.

Too much salt can cause high blood pressure, increasing the risk of heart disease and other health problems. To reduce salt intake, limit the amount added to meals while cooking and at the table.

Choose fresh, natural meals over processed and packaged foods, which are generally rich in salt. Reading food labels and selecting low-sodium or sodium-free options can also make a significant difference.

Recommended servings:

To put these ideas into practice, the DASH Diet recommends serving sizes from various food groups based on calorie levels. These servings provide a flexible framework, allowing people to adjust their diet to their personal needs while remaining true to the essential concepts.

Here are the recommended servings from each food group for a 2,000-calorie DASH diet:

- Grains: 6–8 servings each day. A serving can be 1/2 cup cooked cereal, rice, or pasta, 1 slice of bread, or 1 ounce dry cereal.
- Vegetables: 4–5 servings each day. One serving consists of 1 cup raw leafy green vegetables, 1/2 cup chopped raw or cooked vegetables, or 1/2 cup vegetable juice.
- Fruits: 4-5 servings per day. A serving equals one medium fruit, 1/2 cup fresh, frozen, or canned fruit, or 1/2 cup fruit juice.
- Consume two to three servings of fat-free or low-fat dairy products per day. One serving equals 1 cup of milk or yogurt or One and a half ounces of cheese.
- Lean meats, poultry, and fish: six 1-ounce portions or less each day. One serving equals one ounce of cooked meat, poultry, or fish, or one egg.
- Nuts, seeds, dried beans, and peas: 4 to 5 servings per week. One serving equals 1/3 cup nuts, 2 tablespoons peanut butter, 2 tablespoons seeds, or 1/2 cup cooked dried beans or peas (also known as legumes).

- Fats and oils: 2–3 servings per day. One serving equals one teaspoon of soft margarine, one teaspoon of vegetable oil, one tablespoon of mayonnaise, or two teaspoons of salad dressing.
- Sweets and added sugars: 5 servings or lower per week. One serving equals 1 tablespoon sugar, jelly, or jam, 1/2 cup sorbet, or 1 cup lemonade.

6. Alcohol and Caffeine

Drinking too much alcohol might raise blood pressure. The Dietary Guidelines for Americans recommend that males restrict their alcohol consumption to no more than two drinks per day and women to one or fewer.

The DASH diet does not mention caffeine. Caffeine's effect on blood pressure is unclear. However, caffeine might temporarily increase blood pressure. If you have high blood pressure or believe caffeine impacts your blood pressure, consider cutting back. You might consult your doctor about caffeine.

Take aim at salt!

The foods at the heart of the DASH diet are low in sodium. Following the DASH diet is likely to reduce salt intake.

- To reduce salt, read food labels and choose for low or no-salt-added products.
- Replace salt with salt-free spices or flavorings.
- When cooking rice, pasta, or hot porridge, avoid adding salt.
- Select simple fresh or frozen vegetables.
- Select fresh, skinless poultry, fish, and lean cuts of meat.
- Eat fewer restaurant meals. When dining out, request foods with less salt and ask not to have salt added to your order.

You may find that if you reduce your intake of processed, salty foods, your food tastes differently. Your taste buds may take some time to adjust. But once they do, you might prefer the DASH diet. And you'll be healthier for it.

BENEFITS OF FOLLOWING THE DASH DIET

Now that we've covered the major elements of this heart-healthy diet, let's look at its benefits.

1. Managing blood pressure naturally

The diet's emphasis on fruits and vegetables, whole grains, lean proteins, and low-fat or fat-free dairy foods supports a nutrient-dense eating plan that can naturally lower blood pressure.

According to one study, the DASH diet can naturally lower blood pressure while also preventing or delaying the need for hypertension medication. Another study conducted by the National Heart, Lung, and Blood Institute found that combining this diet with a reduced salt intake decreases blood pressure more than the normal American diet.

2. Reducing the risk of cardiovascular disease

The DASH diet, which contains heart-healthy components, has the potential to drastically lower the risk of heart disease. A study published in the Journal of the American College of Cardiology found that adhering to the diet was connected with a lower risk of developing heart disease, including heart attacks and strokes. Another study found that this diet considerably lowers levels of LDL cholesterol, which is linked to heart disease.

3. Managing and promoting weight loss

The DASH diet can also help you lose and maintain weight over time. It concentrates on fruits, vegetables, whole grains, lean proteins such as chicken or fish, and fat-free dairy products, all of which provide key nutrients yet are low in calories.

The DASH diet also encourages you to watch how much you eat. This implies you consider the size of your meals and respond to your body's signals that it is full. You may lose weight and keep it off for good by eating the correct quantity of food and selecting nutritious options.

4. Increasing insulin sensitivity

Studies have shown that the DASH diet can enhance insulin sensitivity and glucose management. The diet focuses on eating foods rich in blood pressure-lowering substances, which reduces the risk of developing type 2 diabetes. If you already have type 2 diabetes, this diet, like the Mediterranean diet, can help you regulate your blood sugar levels more effectively.

5. Supporting brain health

The diet promotes brain health and cognitive performance. Its emphasis on nutrient-dense foods delivers key vitamins, minerals, and antioxidants required for brain function. According to studies, following the DASH diet may have potential benefits for keeping a healthy brain and lowering the risk of cognitive decline.

6. Increasing energy levels

The DASH diet offers your body with necessary nutrients for healthy energy generation. These meals are high in vitamins, minerals, and fiber, which are essential for sustaining consistent energy throughout the day. Adequate nutritional intake is essential for maintaining your metabolism, which transforms food into energy.

TIPS FOR LONG-TERM SUCCESS

Staying motivated and adhering to the DASH diet are essential components of reaching your health goals. It's extremely important to find a network of friends, family, or even an online community that can encourage and hold you accountable. Surrounding yourself with friendly and encouraging people will help you stay on track and committed to your DASH diet plan.

Another thing to remember is that, in addition to the DASH diet, frequent exercise is an important element of staying healthy. That is why I have included some of the best exercises you can do from the comfort of your home. I recommend starting modestly, such as going for short walks, dancing to your favorite tunes, or playing energetic games with your friends. Then you gradually increase your exercise time, aiming for 150 minutes per week. Combine this healthy diet with exercise and the support of others, and you'll be on your way to a healthier living in no time!

CHAPTER 1

GETTING STARTED WITH THE DASH DIET

Starting the Dietary Approaches to Stop Hypertension (DASH) Diet is a responsible step toward promoting heart health and taking care of your overall well-being. We set the stage for your DASH Diet adventure in this first chapter, offering you in-depth analysis and helpful pointers along the way to a healthier way of living.

FOODS TO FAVOR AND FOODS TO AVOID

1. Fruits:

- Berries (strawberries, blueberries, raspberries)
- Apples
- Oranges
- Bananas
- Mangoes
- Pineapple

2. Vegetables:

- Leafy greens (spinach, kale, collard greens)
- Broccoli
- Carrots
- Bell peppers
- Tomatoes
- Cauliflower

3. Whole Grains:

- Brown rice
- Quinoa

- Oats
- Barley
- Whole wheat pasta
- Bulgur

4. Lean Proteins:

- Skinless poultry (chicken, turkey)
- Lean cuts of beef and pork
- Fish (salmon, trout, tuna)
- Tofu and tempeh
- Legumes (beans, lentils)

5. Nuts, Seeds, and Legumes:

- Almonds
- Walnuts
- Flaxseeds
- Chia seeds
- Lentils
- Chickpeas

6. Dairy:

- Low-fat or fat-free milk

9

- Yogurt
- Cheese (in moderation)

7. Healthy Fats:

- Olive oil
- Avocados
- Nuts and seeds
- Fatty fish (salmon, mackerel)

8. Herbs and Spices:

- Fresh herbs (basil, cilantro, parsley)
- Spices (turmeric, cinnamon, garlic, ginger)
- Vinegar and citrus for flavoring

9. Low-Sodium Foods:

- Fresh or frozen vegetables without added salt
- Unsalted nuts and seeds
- Low-sodium canned beans
- Plain, unsalted popcorn

10. Hydration:

- Water
- Herbal teas
- Infused water with citrus or berries

FOODS TO LIMIT OR AVOID IN THE DASH DIET

1. High-Sodium Foods:

- Processed and packaged foods
- Canned soups and broths
- Deli meats and processed meats
- Salted snacks (chips, pretzels)

2. High-Sugar Foods:

- Sugary beverages (sodas, fruit drinks)
- Candy and sweets
- Pastries and baked goods with added sugars

3. Saturated and Trans Fats:

- Fried foods
- Full-fat dairy products
- Fatty cuts of meat

- Processed snacks high in trans fats

4. Excessive Red Meat:

- Limit red meat intake and choose lean cuts when consumed.

5. High-Fat Dairy:

- Full-fat milk
- Cream
- High-fat cheeses

6. Alcohol:

- If consumed, limit alcoholic beverages. Moderation is key.

7. Added Salt:

- Minimize the use of table salt and limit high-sodium condiments.

8. Sugary Beverages:

- Limit or avoid sugary drinks, opting for water or unsweetened beverages.

By favoring nutrient-dense foods and being mindful of sodium and sugar intake, you can tailor your diet to align with the principles of the DASH Diet, promoting heart health and overall well-being.

GROCERY SHOPPING FOR DASH DIET

Buying on the DASH Diet is not that difficult. Your neighborhood store has everything you could possibly need. To check for excessive fat or high sodium intake, you should learn to read nutrition labels.

- Low-fat, low-sodium beef, and poultry
- Fruit: citrus, apples, mangoes, pineapple, bananas, berries, and citrus
- Vegetables, such as potatoes, carrots, broccoli, asparagus, cucumbers, and greens.
- Eggs
- Halibut, trout, and salmon
- Sunflower seeds, walnuts, and almonds

- Low-fat plain yogurt

SODIUM

Your objective when following the DASH Diet is to cut back on sodium to 2,300 mg daily. After you achieve that dosage, discuss with your physician cutting it down to 1,500 mg daily. Approximately 3,400 mg of sodium are consumed daily by most Americans. The sodium in processed foods is mostly responsible for that.

There are two methods to search for foods with reduced salt content when following the DASH Diet. To start, you can check the product's salt content by reading the labels on the front of the packaging. The meanings of different expressions vary.

- A food item labeled as sodium- or salt-free has fewer than five milligrams of sodium per serving.
- A food item designated as "very low sodium" has 35 mg of sodium or less per serving.
- A food item is considered low sodium if each serving has 140 milligrams or less of salt.
- A serving of 3-1/2 ounces (100 grams) of a low-sodium meal has 140 mg of sodium or less.
- Light in sodium refers to a food that has 50% less sodium than its standard counterpart.
- If a product is labeled as unsalted or has no added salt, it does not mean that salt was added during processing; it is not a sodium-free food.

Examining the Nutrition Facts label is another method to determine salt content. Sodium is listed underneath cholesterol in the middle of the label. Make an effort to select foods that have less than 5% of the recommended daily intake of salt. High-sodium foods are those that contain 20% or more of the recommended daily intake of salt.

Generally speaking, choose fresh, frozen, or plain veggies as they typically have less sodium than canned foods. Always give canned veggies a thorough rinsing. By doing this, the sodium is reduced by around half.

Fish, skinless chicken, and lean meat pieces that are fresh or frozen have less sodium than those that are canned, smoked, brined, or cured. Finally, check the labels of baked items (such as bread and crackers), salad dressing, sauces, and even processed cheese. Unexpectedly, several of these foods are high in salt.

Finally, go down the nutrition label to see how much potassium is in the meal while you're checking it for sodium. The goal of the DASH Diet is to increase the impact of lowering blood pressure by assisting you in achieving a daily target of 4,700 milligrams of potassium. Potatoes, bananas, yogurt, lima beans, and orange juice are foods high in potassium.

FAT

On the DASH Diet, you will also consume less fat. You will naturally consume less fatty foods as you increase your consumption of fruits and veggies. To achieve your objectives, you can select lower-fat foods when you go grocery shopping.

Once more, read labels to choose healthier foods. Phrases that appear on labels have distinct meanings.

- A food item is considered fat-free if it has fewer than 0.5 grams of fat per serving.
- A food item is considered low in saturated fat if it has one gram or less of saturated fat per serving and 15% or fewer calories from saturated fat.
- A food item is considered low-fat if it has three grams or fewer per serving.
- If a dish is considered "light in fat," it signifies that it only has half as much fat as the original.

These front-label statements, meanwhile, don't often accurately reflect the food's true worth. Not all foods without fat are good for you. When fat is eliminated, sugars or carbs are frequently added to make up for it. Furthermore, not all fat is made equal. Mono- and polyunsaturated fats are examples of unsaturated fats that are beneficial to consume in moderation.

Finding naturally fat-free or low-fat products may become easier as you grow used to shopping the perimeter (outside ring) of the supermarket for DASH-friendly foods. Additionally, you'll notice that certain foods are lower in salt.

While there are no items that are forbidden on the DASH Diet, you will discover that eating meals that are minimally processed and as close to their entire form can allow you to have more fulfilling meals.

First, put fruits, vegetables, and whole grains in your shopping basket. Next, make a smaller area for dairy products that are low in fat and/or include lean protein. Nuts, seeds, candies, fats, and oils should occupy very little space in your basket because they are restricted items on the diet.

HOW TO READ LABELS

Almost all food products have nutrition labels, sometimes known as nutrition facts panels. Take the product from the shelf at the grocery store and turn it to the right to see the nutrition label. When there is no right side, as in the case of a flexible pouch, the nutrition label is the sole instance in which it is not to the right of the main display panel. The nutritional data is then located on the reverse side.

A brief nutritional summary of the food is given to the consumer by nutrition labels. Labels are made to be user-friendly and easy for customers to read. However, diet is a complicated topic. Nutrition labels are not the simplest tables to read, despite their best efforts to be clear.

Based On A Diet Of 2000 Calories

Most labels have a footnote at the bottom with the nutrition label key. "The percent daily values are predicated on a diet of 2000 calories.," it says. It adheres to that recommendation even in the event that the footnote is absent from the nutrition label. There simply isn't enough space in certain packages to include it.

Every daily percentage number is predicated on a 2000 calorie intake. It was intended to assist people. Customers only need to aim for 100% of each nutrient in a day rather than remembering how much to eat of each one. In the unlikely event that the 2000-calorie diet does not apply, all of the nutrients are also stated in grams or milligrams.

This additional resource will assist you in learning how to read the labels on any product.

SCAN THIS IMAGE TO DOWNLOAD RESOURCE

ADDITIONAL INFORMATION

The content and arrangement of nutrition labels are required by law. The mandatory components are indicated by the labels in this post. Some elements are optional, such as polyunsaturated and monounsaturated fatty acids and sugar alcohols. Other ingredients are expressly prohibited, such as amino acids. There are standards for determining calories and percentage daily values, but that is a topic for another discussion.

Even the label's appearance is restricted. Type size and line spacing must be within a particular range, upper and lower-case characters are required, and some elements must be bold. These are only just a few of the standards.

As you can see, the government views food labels as vital. Mistakes can cost a corporation a lot of money in fines and reprinting fees. Because firms seek to avoid these fines, many create positions that only focus on labels. These professionals ensure that nutrition labels fulfill all rules.

As we complete this chapter, you've taken the critical initial steps toward creating a health-conscious lifestyle. By delving into the details of which foods to prefer and which to avoid, you've not only got a solid comprehension of the DASH Diet but also the wisdom to make informed dietary decisions.

You've embraced the essence of the DASH Diet by walking the aisles of your grocery store with a planned shopping list in hand. Each chosen item becomes a source of nourishment, adding to a culinary palette that values freshness, balance, and nutritional depth. Your journey goes beyond the act of buying; it is a conscious investment in your well-being.

Furthermore, reading the language of nutrition labels has given you a skill that goes beyond the confines of the supermarket. It's a tool that helps you negotiate the intricacies of packaged foods, ensuring that every addition to your pantry adheres to the principles of heart-healthy living. As you carry these insights forward, imagine a kitchen converted into a health sanctuary, with each meal serving as more than just food but also a conscious act of self-care.

The upcoming chapters promise delectable recipes, practical culinary wisdom, and a holistic approach that extends beyond the kitchen. Your journey, full of potential and purpose, has only just begun, and the DASH Diet will be your constant companion on the route to a healthier, more vibrant version of yourself. Moving on to the next chapter, a blank canvas waiting for your culinary inventiveness and well-being.

CHAPTER 2

BREAKFAST RECIPES

1. SWEET POTATO HASH BROWNS

Cook time: 30 mins   **Yield**: 4

Ingredients

- 2 medium-sized sweet potatoes, peeled and grated
- 1 small onion, finely chopped
- 2 tablespoons olive oil
- Salt and pepper to taste
- 1 teaspoon paprika (optional)

Instructions

- Preheat a skillet over medium heat and add olive oil.
- In a bowl, combine grated sweet potatoes, chopped onion, salt, pepper, and paprika.
- Form small patties from the mixture and place them in the skillet.
- Allow to cook for approximately ten minutes on both sides, till they're crisp and golden.
- Serve hot and enjoy the classic goodness of sweet potato hash browns.

Nutritional Facts: Calories: 150, Protein: 2g, Carbohydrates: 25g, Fiber: 4g, Fat: 5g, Saturated Fat: 1g, Sodium: 220mg

2. QUINOA FRUIT SALAD

Cook time:30 mins   **Yield**: 4

Ingredients

- 1 cup quinoa, cooked and cooled
- 1 cup strawberries, sliced
- 1 cup blueberries
- 1 cup pineapple, diced
- 1/2 cup fresh mint leaves, chopped
- 2 tablespoons honey
- 1 tablespoon olive oil
- 1 tablespoon fresh lime juice

Instructions

- In a large bowl, combine cooked quinoa, strawberries, blueberries, pineapple, and mint.
- In a separate small bowl, whisk together honey, olive oil, and lime juice.
- Pour the dressing over the quinoa and fruit mixture, tossing gently to coat.
- Before serving, let the food cool in the fridge for a minimum of fifteen minutes.
- Garnish with additional mint leaves if desired and enjoy this refreshing quinoa fruit salad.

Nutritional Facts: Calories: 220, Protein: 5g, Carbohydrates: 40g, Fiber: 5g, Fat: 5g, Saturated Fat: 1g, Sodium: 10mg

3. COTTAGE CHEESE WITH FRUITS

Cook time: 10 mins   **Yield:** 2

Ingredients

- 1 cup low-fat cottage cheese
- 1 cup mixed fruits (such as berries, peaches, and kiwi), diced
- 1 tablespoon honey
- 2 tablespoons chopped nuts (almonds, walnuts, or pistachios)

Instructions

- In individual serving bowls, spoon half a cup of cottage cheese.
- Top with mixed fruits and drizzle honey over the fruits.
- Sprinkle chopped nuts on top for added crunch and nutritional benefits.
- Repeat for the second serving.
- Serve chilled and relish this delightful and nutritious cottage cheese with fruits..

Nutritional Facts: Calories: 220, Protein: 16g, Carbohydrates: 25g, Fiber: 4g, Fat: 8g, Saturated Fat: 2g, Sodium: 350mg

4. YOGURT WITH GRANOLA AND FRUIT

Cook time: 10 mins   **Yield:** 2

Ingredients

- 1 cup low-fat Greek yogurt
- 1/2 cup granola (choose a low-sugar option)
- 1 cup mixed berries (strawberries, blueberries, raspberries)
- 1 tablespoon honey

Instructions

- In individual bowls, spoon half a cup of Greek yogurt.
- Top with granola and mixed berries.
- Drizzle honey over the yogurt, granola, and berries.
- Repeat for the second serving.
- Serve chilled and enjoy this delightful and nutritious Yogurt With Granola and Fruit.

Nutritional Facts: Calories: 250, Protein: 14g, Carbohydrates: 42g, Fiber: 6g, Fat: 5g, Saturated Fat: 1g, Sodium: 80mg

5. QUINOA BREAKFAST PORRIDGE WITH ALMOND BUTTER

Cook time:20 mins   **Yield:** 2

Ingredients

- 1/2 cup quinoa, rinsed
- 1 cup almond milk
- 1 ripe banana, mashed
- 1 tablespoon almond butter
- 1/2 teaspoon cinnamon
- Fresh berries for topping

Instructions

- In a saucepan, combine quinoa and almond milk. Bring to a boil, then reduce heat and simmer until quinoa is cooked and the mixture thickens.

- Stir in mashed banana, almond butter, and cinnamon.

- Continue cooking for an additional 5 minutes, stirring frequently.

- Divide into bowls, top with fresh berries, and savor this wholesome Quinoa Breakfast Porridge.

Nutritional Facts: Calories: 320, Protein: 9g, Carbohydrates: 55g, Fiber: 7g, Fat: 8g, Saturated Fat: 1g, Sodium: 80mg

6. BANANA AND SPINACH SMOOTHIES

Cook time: 10 mins   **Yield: 2**

Ingredients

- 2 ripe bananas
- 2 cups fresh spinach leaves
- 1 cup low-fat Greek yogurt
- 1/2 cup almond milk
- 1 tablespoon chia seeds
- Ice cubes (optional)
- Honey or maple syrup to taste

Instructions

- In a blender, combine bananas, spinach, Greek yogurt, almond milk, and chia seeds.

- Blend until smooth. Add ice cubes if a colder consistency is desired.

- Taste and sweeten with honey or maple syrup as needed.

- Pour into glasses and enjoy this nutrient-packed Banana and Spinach Smoothie.

Nutritional Facts: Calories: 180, Protein: 8g, Carbohydrates: 30g, Fiber: 6g, Fat: 4g, Saturated Fat: 1g, Sodium: 60mg

7. BERRY AND SPINACH SALAD

Prep time: 15 mins   **Yield: 4**

Ingredients

- 4 cups fresh spinach leaves
- 1 cup mixed berries (strawberries, blueberries, raspberries)
- 1/2 cup sliced cucumber
- 1/4 cup crumbled feta cheese
- 1/4 cup chopped walnuts
- 2 tablespoons balsamic vinaigrette dressing
- Salt and pepper to taste

Instructions

- In a large bowl, combine fresh spinach, mixed berries, sliced cucumber, crumbled feta cheese, and chopped walnuts.
- Drizzle balsamic vinaigrette dressing over the salad.
- Toss gently to coat all ingredients evenly.
- Season with salt and pepper to taste.
- Serve immediately, enjoying the vibrant flavors of this Berry and Spinach Salad.

Nutritional Facts: 120 calories, 5g protein, 10g carbohydrates, 7g fat, 1.5g saturated fat, 180mg sodium

8. BANANA WALNUT MUFFINS

Total Cooking time: 35 mins   Yield: 12

Ingredients

- 2 ripe bananas, mashed
- 1/2 cup unsweetened applesauce
- 1/4 cup honey
- 1/4 cup olive oil
- 2 large eggs
- 1 teaspoon vanilla extract
- 2 cups whole wheat flour
- 1 teaspoon baking soda
- 1/2 teaspoon cinnamon
- 1/4 teaspoon salt
- 1/2 cup chopped walnuts

Instructions

- Preheat oven to 350°F (175°C). Put paper liners inside a muffin tin.
- In a large bowl, mix mashed bananas, applesauce, honey, olive oil, eggs, and vanilla extract.
- In a separate bowl, whisk together whole wheat flour, baking soda, cinnamon, and salt.
- Stirring until just blended, gradually add the dry ingredients to the banana mixture.
- Add the chopped walnuts and fold.
- Pour the batter into each muffin cup, filling it to approximately two thirds of the way.
- When a toothpick put into the center comes out clean, bake for 18 to 20 minutes.
- Allow muffins to cool before serving.

Nutritional Facts: 160 calories, 3g protein, 22g carbohydrates, 7g fat, 1g saturated fat, 130mg sodium

9. VEGGIE FRITTATA WITH HERBS

Cooking time: 30 mins   **Yield: 4**

Ingredients

- 6 large eggs
- 1/2 cup skim milk
- 1 cup cherry tomatoes, halved

- 1/2 cup bell peppers, diced
- 1/2 cup zucchini, sliced
- 1/4 cup red onion, finely chopped
- 2 tablespoons fresh herbs (such as parsley, chives, or dill), chopped
- Salt and pepper to taste
- 1 tablespoon olive oil

Instructions

- Preheat the oven to 375°F (190°C).
- In a bowl, whisk together eggs and skim milk. Season with salt and pepper.
- In a skillet that is oven safe, warm the olive oil over medium heat.
- Red onion, bell peppers, zucchini, and cherry tomatoes should all be added to the skillet. Cook until veggies are tender, about 5 minutes.
- Cover the veggies with the egg mixture.
- Add some fresh herbs on the top.
- After transferring the skillet to the preheated oven, bake the frittata for 15 minutes, or until it sets.
- Slice and serve warm.

Nutritional Facts: 180 calories, 12g protein, 8g carbohydrates, 11g fat, 2.5g saturated fat, 320mg sodium

10.   HOMEMADE MUESLI

Cooking time: 15 mins   **Yield:** 2

Ingredients

- 4 large eggs
- 1 cup fresh spinach, chopped
- 1/4 cup crumbled feta cheese
- 1 tablespoon olive oil
- Salt and pepper to taste
- Fresh herbs (optional, for garnish)

Instructions

- In a bowl, whisk together eggs, chopped spinach, and crumbled feta. Season with salt and pepper.
- Heat olive oil in the non-stick skillet over medium heat.
- Once the egg mixture is in the skillet, cook it over low heat, stirring occasionally, until the eggs set.
- Garnish with fresh herbs if desired.
- Serve hot and savor this nutritious Scrambled Eggs With Spinach and Feta.

Nutritional Facts: 220 calories, 15g protein, 5g carbohydrates, 16g fat, 6g saturated fat, 350mg sodium

11.   TOFU SCRAMBLE

Cooking time: 25 mins   **Yield:** 2

Ingredients

- 1 block firm tofu, crumbled
- 1 cup bell peppers, diced
- 1/2 cup cherry tomatoes, halved

- 1/4 cup red onion, finely chopped
- 2 cloves garlic, minced
- 1 tablespoon nutritional yeast
- 1 teaspoon turmeric
- Salt and pepper to taste
- 1 tablespoon olive oil

Instructions

- In a skillet over medium heat, warm the olive oil. Add red onion and garlic, and sauté until softened.
- Add crumbled tofu, bell peppers, cherry tomatoes, nutritional yeast, turmeric, salt, and pepper.
- Cook, stirring occasionally, until tofu is heated through and vegetables are tender.
- Adjust seasoning if needed.
- Serve warm and relish the flavors of this plant-based Tofu Scramble..

Nutritional Facts: 230 calories, 16g protein, 10g carbohydrates, 15g fat, 2g saturated fat, 380mg sodium

12. BLUEBERRY AND ALMOND OVERNIGHT OATS

Cooking time: 8hrs 5mins   **Yield:** 2
Ingredients

- 1 cup old-fashioned oats
- 1 cup unsweetened almond milk
- 1/2 cup fresh blueberries

- 2 tablespoons almond butter
- 1 tablespoon chia seeds
- 1 tablespoon maple syrup
- 1/2 teaspoon vanilla extract

Instructions

- In a jar or bowl, combine oats, almond milk, blueberries, almond butter, chia seeds, maple syrup, and vanilla extract.
- Make sure that every single ingredien is well combined by giving it a good stir.
- For the entire night, cover and chill.
- Stir the oats thoroughly in the morning.
- Serve chilled and enjoy these delightful Blueberry and Almond Overnight Oats.

Nutritional Facts: 320 calories, 9g protein, 45g carbohydrates, 12g fat, 1g saturated fat, 90mg sodium

13. OATMEAL WITH MIXED BERRIES

Cooking time: 10 mins   **Yield:** 2

Ingredients

- 1 cup old-fashioned oats
- 2 cups water or low-fat milk
- 1 cup mixed berries (strawberries, blueberries, raspberries)
- 1 tablespoon chia seeds

- 1 tablespoon honey or maple syrup
- 1/4 cup chopped nuts (almonds, walnuts)
- Cinnamon for garnish (optional)

Instructions

- Heat up some milk or water in a saucepan.
- Add the oats and turn down the heat. Simmer for roughly five minutes, stirring now and then.
- Take off the heat and mix in chopped nuts, honey or maple syrup, chia seeds, and assorted berries.
- Give it a minute to settle so the flavors can combine.
- If preferred, add a dash of cinnamon as a garnish.
- Serve warm and relish the goodness of this DASH Diet Oatmeal With Mixed Berries.

Nutritional Information (per serving): 280 calories, 9g protein, 45g carbohydrates, 9g fat, 1g saturated fat, 60mg sodium

- 1/4 cup fresh basil leaves, chopped
- Salt and pepper to taste
- 2 tablespoons olive oil
- 1/4 cup feta cheese, crumbled (optional)

Instructions

- In a bowl, whisk together eggs, cherry tomatoes, basil, salt, and pepper.
- In a nonstick skillet set over medium heat, warm the olive oil.
- After adding the egg mixture to the skillet, heat it until the edges are firm.
- Gently lift the edges with a spatula, allowing uncooked eggs to flow underneath.
- When the omelet is mostly set, sprinkle crumbled feta cheese if desired.
- Fold the omelet in half and serve hot.
- Enjoy the freshness of this DASH Diet Tomatoes and Basil Omelet..

Nutritional Facts: 240 calories, 12g protein, 5g carbohydrates, 18g fat, 5g saturated fat, 350mg sodium

14. TOMATOES AND BASIL OMELETS

Cooking time: 10 mins   **Yield:** 2

Ingredients

- 4 large eggs
- 1 cup cherry tomatoes, halved

15. VEGGIE AND HUMMUS WRAP

Cooking time: 10 mins   **Yield:** 2

Ingredients

- Three bell peppers, green
- 2 whole-grain wraps

- 1 cup mixed vegetables (bell peppers, cucumbers, tomatoes), thinly sliced
- 1/2 cup hummus
- 1/4 cup feta cheese, crumbled
- Parsley or cilantro, or other fresh herbs, to garnish

Instructions

- Lay out the wraps and spread a generous layer of hummus on each.
- Divide the mixed vegetables evenly between the wraps.
- Sprinkle crumbled feta cheese on top of the vegetables.
- Garnish with fresh herbs.
- Fold in the sides and roll up each wrap.
- Slice in half and serve these delightful DASH Diet Veggie and Hummus Wraps.

Nutritional information: 330 calories, 11g protein, 45g carbohydrates, 13g fat, 3g saturated fat, 480mg sodium

16. CHICKEN EGG WRAPS

Cooking time: 20 mins   **Yield:** 2

Ingredients

- 2 whole-grain wraps
- 1 cup cooked chicken breast, shredded
- 2 large eggs, scrambled
- 1 cup mixed vegetables (bell peppers, spinach, onions), sautéed

- 1/4 cup salsa
- Salt and pepper to taste
- Fresh cilantro for garnish (optional)

Instructions

- In a skillet, sauté mixed vegetables until tender.
- Add shredded chicken and scrambled eggs to the skillet. Cook until eggs are set.
- Season with salt and pepper to taste.
- Lay out the wraps and spoon the chicken and egg mixture onto each.
- Top with salsa and garnish with fresh cilantro if desired.
- Roll up the wraps, slice in half, and serve these hearty DASH Diet Chicken Egg Wraps.

Nutritional Facts: 380 calories, 32g protein, 30g carbohydrates, 15g fat, 3g saturated fat, 630mg sodium

17. SAUTEED MUSHROOMS WITH EGG

Cooking time: 15 mins   **Yield:** 5

Ingredients

- 2 cups mushrooms, sliced
- 2 large eggs
- 1 tablespoon olive oil
- 2 cloves garlic, minced
- 1 tablespoon fresh parsley, chopped

- Salt and pepper to taste
- Whole-grain toast for serving

Instructions

- In a skillet over medium heat, warm the olive oil. When aromatic, add the minced garlic and sauté it.
- Sliced mushrooms should be added and cooked until they release moisture and turn golden.
- In each mushroom well, make a well and crack an egg into it.
- Cook the eggs until they reach your desired doneness.
- Season with salt, pepper, and fresh parsley.
- Serve over whole-grain toast and enjoy this savory DASH Diet Sauteed Mushrooms With Egg..

Nutritional Facts: 220 calories, 12g protein, 10g carbohydrates, 15g fat, 3g saturated fat, 160mg sodium

18.   BULLET COFFEE

Cooking time: 5 mins   **Yield:** 1

Ingredients

- 1 cup brewed coffee
- 1 tablespoon unsalted butter
- 1 tablespoon coconut oil or MCT oil
- 1 tablespoon heavy cream
- Stevia or your preferred sweetener (optional)

Instructions

- Brew a cup of coffee.
- In a blender, combine brewed coffee, unsalted butter, coconut oil or MCT oil, and heavy cream.
- Blend until frothy and well combined.
- Add sweetener if desired, and blend again.
- Pour into a mug and savor this energizing DASH Diet Bullet Coffee.

Nutritional Facts: 210 calories, 0g protein, 0g carbohydrates, 24g fat, 18g saturated fat, 10mg sodium

19.   APPLE OATS

Cooking time: 10 mins   **Yield: 2**

Ingredients

- 1 cup old-fashioned oats
- 2 cups water or low-fat milk
- 1 apple, diced
- 1 tablespoon almond butter
- 1 tablespoon chia seeds
- Cinnamon and nutmeg to taste
- 1 tablespoon honey or maple syrup (optional)

Instructions

- Heat up some milk or water in a pot.

- Add the oats and turn down the heat. Simmer for roughly five minutes, stirring now and then.
- Stir in diced apple, almond butter, chia seeds, cinnamon, nutmeg, and sweetener if desired.
- Let it sit for a minute to allow flavors to meld.
- Serve warm and enjoy the comforting goodness of DASH Diet Apple Oats..

Nutritional Facts: 280 calories, 8g protein, 45g carbohydrates, 8g fat, 1g saturated fat, 60mg sodium

20. CHEESE PANINI

Cooking time: 10 mins   **Yield:** 2

Ingredients

- 4 slices whole-grain bread
- 1 cup low-fat mozzarella cheese, shredded
- 1 tomato, sliced
- Fresh basil leaves
- Olive oil cooking spray

Instructions

- Preheat a panini press or skillet.
- On each slice of bread, layer mozzarella cheese, tomato slices, and fresh basil.
- Top with the remaining bread slices to form sandwiches.

- Lightly spray the outer sides of the sandwiches with olive oil cooking spray.
- Grill in the panini press or skillet until the cheese melts and the bread is golden brown.
- Slice and serve these delicious DASH Diet Cheese Paninis.

Nutritional Facts: 330 calories, 18g protein, 40g carbohydrates, 12g fat, 5g saturated fat, 450mg sodium

21. QUARK SANDWICH

Cooking time: 10 mins   **Yield:** 2

Ingredients

- 4 slices whole-grain bread
- 1 cup quark cheese
- 1 cucumber, thinly sliced
- 1/2 red onion, thinly sliced
- 1 tablespoon fresh dill, chopped
- Salt and pepper to taste

Instructions

- Spread quark cheese evenly on each slice of bread.
- Layer cucumber slices and red onion on two slices of bread.
- Sprinkle with fresh dill and season with salt and pepper.
- To make sandwiches, place the remaining bread slices on top.

- Slice and serve these refreshing DASH Diet Quark Sandwiches.

Nutritional Facts: 280 calories, 14g protein, 45g carbohydrates, 6g fat, 1.5g saturated fat, 400mg sodium

22. BROCCOLI CHEESE EGG MUFFINS

Cooking time: 30 mins   **Yield:** 6

Ingredients

- 6 large eggs
- 1 cup broccoli florets, finely chopped
- 1/2 cup shredded cheddar cheese
- 1/4 cup milk (low-fat)
- 1/2 teaspoon garlic powder
- Salt and pepper to taste
- Cooking spray

Instructions

- Preheat the oven to 375°F (190°C). Use cooking spray to grease a muffin tray.
- In a bowl, whisk together eggs, milk, garlic powder, salt, and pepper.
- Divide chopped broccoli evenly among the muffin cups.
- Pour the egg mixture over the broccoli in each cup.
- Sprinkle shredded cheddar cheese on top.

- Bake for 20 minutes or until the eggs are set and the tops are golden.
- Let cool slightly before taking them out of the tin.
- Serve and relish these tasty DASH Diet Broccoli Cheese Egg Muffins.

Nutritional Facts: 140 calories, 11g protein, 3g carbohydrates, 9g fat, 3.5g saturated fat, 180mg sodium

23. HARD-BOILED EGGS

Cooking time: 13 mins   **Yield:** 4

Ingredients

- 4 large eggs

Instructions

- Put the eggs in a saucepan in a single layer.
- Make sure the eggs are submerged by adding water to the cover.
- Put the water on medium-high heat and bring it to a boil.
- Once boiling, reduce the heat to low, cover, and simmer for 12 minutes.
- Transfer eggs to an ice bath to cool quickly.
- Peel and sprinkle with a pinch of salt if desired.
- Enjoy these simple and protein-packed DASH Diet Hard-Boiled Eggs.

Nutritional Facts: 70 calories, 6g protein, 0g carbohydrates, 5g fat, 1.5g saturated fat, 70mg sodium

Nutritional Facts: 250 calories, 10g protein, 10g carbohydrates, 20g fat, 4g saturated fat, 120mg sodium

24. BAKED AVOCADO EGGS

Cooking time: 20 mins   **Yield:** 2

Ingredients

- 1 avocado, halved and pitted
- 2 eggs
- Salt and pepper to taste
- For garnish, use fresh herbs like parsley or chives

Instructions

- Preheat the oven to 375°F (190°C).
- Scoop out a small portion of the avocado flesh to make room for the egg.
- Place the avocado halves in a baking dish to prevent tipping.
- Crack an egg into each avocado half.
- Sprinkle with salt and pepper.
- Bake until the eggs are cooked to your desired consistency, around 15 minutes.
- Garnish with fresh herbs.
- Serve and savor these creamy and nutritious DASH Diet Baked Avocado Eggs.

25. PEACH PANCAKES

Cooking time: 25 mins   **Yield:** 4

Ingredients

- 1 cup whole-wheat flour
- 1 tablespoon baking powder
- 1/2 teaspoon cinnamon
- 1 cup low-fat milk
- 1 large egg
- 2 tablespoons olive oil
- 1 peach, peeled and diced
- Cooking spray

Instructions

- In a bowl, whisk together whole-wheat flour, baking powder, and cinnamon.
- Combine the whole-wheat flour, cinnamon, and baking powder in a bowl.
- Whisk together the egg, olive oil, and milk in a separate bowl.
- Stir just until mixed after adding the wet components to the dry ingredients.
- Add the diced peach and fold gently.
- Coat with cooking spray and preheat a nonstick skillet or griddle over medium heat.
- Transfer 1/4 cup of batter onto the griddle for every pancake.

- Simmer until surface bubbles appear, then turn and continue cooking until the other side becomes golden brown.
- Serve warm and enjoy these delightful DASH Diet Peach Pancakes.

Nutritional Facts: 200 calories, 7g protein, 30g carbohydrates, 7g fat, 1g saturated fat, 250mg sodium

CHAPTER 3

LUNCH RECIPES

26. BAKED SALMON WITH ROASTED VEGETABLES

Cooking time: 40 mins   **Yield:** 2

Ingredients

- 2 salmon fillets
- Two cups of mixed veggies, including cherry tomatoes, zucchini, and bell peppers
- 1 tablespoon olive oil
- 1 teaspoon garlic powder
- 1 teaspoon dried oregano
- Salt and pepper to taste
- Lemon wedges for serving

Instructions

- Preheat the oven to 400°F (200°C).
- Arrange the salmon fillets on a parchment paper-lined baking pan.
- Mix together mixed vegetables, salt, pepper, dried oregano, and olive oil.
- Arrange the veggies on the baking sheet in a circle around the salmon.
- Bake for 20-25 minutes or until the salmon is cooked through and the vegetables are tender.
- Serve with lemon wedges and relish this nutritious DASH Diet Baked Salmon With Roasted Vegetables.

Nutritional Facts: 350 calories, 30g protein, 15g carbohydrates, 20g fat, 3g saturated fat, 400mg sodium

27. GREEK-STYLE QUINOA SALAD

Cooking time: 20 mins   **Yield:** 4

Ingredients

- 1 cup quinoa, cooked and cooled
- 1 cucumber, diced
- 1 cup cherry tomatoes, halved
- 1/2 cup Kalamata olives, sliced
- 1/4 cup red onion, finely chopped
- 1/2 cup feta cheese, crumbled
- 2 tablespoons olive oil
- 1 tablespoon red wine vinegar
- 1 teaspoon dried oregano
- Salt and pepper to taste

Instructions

- In a large bowl, combine cooked quinoa, cucumber, cherry tomatoes, Kalamata olives, red onion, and feta cheese.
- Mix the olive oil, red wine vinegar, dried oregano, salt, and pepper in a small bowl.

- After adding the dressing to the quinoa mixture, toss to blend.
- Serve chilled and enjoy the vibrant flavors of this DASH Diet Greek-Style Quinoa Salad.
- **Nutritional Facts:** 320 calories, 10g protein, 35g carbohydrates, 16g fat, 5g saturated fat, 450mg sodium

28. VEGETABLE STIR-FRY WITH BROWN RICE

Cooking time: 35 mins   **Yield:** 4

Ingredients

- 2 cups broccoli florets
- 1 cup snap peas, trimmed
- 1 red bell pepper, sliced
- 1 carrot, julienned
- 2 tablespoons low-sodium soy sauce
- 1 tablespoon sesame oil
- 1 tablespoon olive oil
- 1 teaspoon ginger, grated
- 2 cloves garlic, minced
- 2 cups cooked brown rice

Instructions

- Olive and sesame oils should be heated over medium-high heat in a wok or big pan.
- Add ginger and garlic, stir-fry for 30 seconds.

- Add broccoli, snap peas, red bell pepper, and carrot. Stir-fry for 5-7 minutes until vegetables are tender-crisp.
- Pour in low-sodium soy sauce and toss to coat.
- Serve the stir-fried vegetables over cooked brown rice.
- Enjoy this wholesome DASH Diet Vegetable Stir-fry With Brown Rice.

Nutritional Facts: 280 calories, 8g protein, 40g carbohydrates, 10g fat, 2g saturated fat, 500mg sodium

29. SHRIMP AND AVOCADO SALAD

Cooking time: 23 mins + 1hr   **Yield:** 4

Ingredients

- 1 pound shrimp, peeled and deveined
- 2 avocados, diced
- 2 cups mixed salad greens
- 1 cup cherry tomatoes, halved
- 1/4 cup red onion, thinly sliced
- 1/4 cup cilantro, chopped
- 1 tablespoon olive oil
- 1 tablespoon lime juice
- Salt and pepper to taste

Instructions

- Season shrimp with salt and pepper.

- Olive oil should be heated in a skillet over medium-high heat. Cook shrimp for 2-3 minutes per side until opaque.
- In a large bowl, combine salad greens, diced avocados, cherry tomatoes, red onion, and cilantro.
- Add cooked shrimp to the salad.
- Drizzle with lime juice, toss gently to combine.
- Serve immediately and savor the freshness of this DASH Diet Shrimp and Avocado Salad.

Nutritional Facts: 350 calories, 30g protein, 15g carbohydrates, 20g fat, 3g saturated fat, 400mg sodium

30.   GRILLED SHRIMP WITH VEGETABLE KABOBS

Cooking time: 30 mins   **Yield:** 4

Ingredients

- 1 pound large shrimp, peeled and deveined
- 2 zucchini, sliced
- 1 red bell pepper, cut into chunks
- 1 yellow bell pepper, cut into chunks
- 1 red onion, cut into wedges
- 2 tablespoons olive oil
- 1 tablespoon lemon juice
- 1 teaspoon dried oregano
- Salt and pepper to taste

Instructions

- Preheat the grill to medium-high heat.
- In a bowl, toss shrimp, zucchini, bell peppers, and red onion with olive oil, lemon juice, dried oregano, salt, and pepper.
- Thread shrimp and vegetables onto skewers.
- Grill for 3-4 minutes per side until shrimp are opaque and vegetables are tender.
- Serve these flavorful DASH Diet Grilled Shrimp with Vegetable Kabobs.
- **Nutritional Facts:** 280 calories, 25g protein, 15g carbohydrates, 14g fat, 2g saturated fat, 400mg sodium

31.   BAKED CHICKEN AND VEGETABLE FOIL PACKETS

Cooking time: 40mins   **Yield:** 2

Ingredients

- 2 boneless, skinless chicken breasts
- 2 cups broccoli florets
- 1 bell pepper, sliced
- 1 carrot, julienned
- 2 tablespoons olive oil
- 1 teaspoon Italian seasoning
- Salt and pepper to taste
- Lemon slices for garnish

Instructions

- Preheat the oven to 400°F (200°C).
- Place each chicken breast on a large piece of foil.
- Surround each chicken breast with broccoli, bell pepper, and julienned carrot.
- Drizzle olive oil over each chicken and vegetable packet.
- Sprinkle with Italian seasoning, salt, and pepper.
- Place the sealed foil packets on a baking sheet.
- Bake for 25 minutes or until the chicken is cooked through.
- Garnish with lemon slices and serve these delicious DASH Diet Baked Chicken and Vegetable Foil Packets.

Nutritional Facts: 320 calories, 30g protein, 15g carbohydrates, 16g fat, 3g saturated fat, 400mg sodium

32. TURKEY AND VEGETABLE CHILI

Cooking time: 45 mins   **Yield:** 4

Ingredients

- 1 pound lean ground turkey
- 1 onion, diced
- 2 bell peppers, diced
- 2 cloves garlic, minced
- One can (15 oz) of washed and drained kidney beans

- 1 can (15 oz) diced tomatoes
- 1 cup corn kernels (fresh or frozen)
- 1 cup low-sodium vegetable broth
- 2 tablespoons chili powder
- 1 teaspoon cumin
- Salt and pepper to taste
- Fresh cilantro for garnish

Instructions

- Brown the ground turkey over medium heat in a big saucepan.
- Add diced onion, bell peppers, and minced garlic. Sauté until vegetables are softened.
- Stir in kidney beans, diced tomatoes, corn, vegetable broth, chili powder, cumin, salt, and pepper.
- Bring to a simmer and let it cook for 20-25 minutes, stirring occasionally.
- Adjust seasoning if needed.
- Serve hot, garnished with fresh cilantro.
- Enjoy this hearty and flavorful DASH Diet Turkey and Vegetable Chili.

Nutritional Facts: 320 calories, 25g protein, 30g carbohydrates, 10g fat, 3g saturated fat, 500mg sodium

33. QUINOA AND SPINACH STUFFED PEPPERS

Cooking time: 40 mins   **Yield:** 4

Ingredients

- 4 bell peppers, halved and seeds removed
- 1 cup quinoa, cooked
- 2 cups fresh spinach, chopped
- One can (15 oz) of rinsed and drained black beans
- 1 cup corn kernels (fresh or frozen)
- 1 cup tomato sauce
- 1 teaspoon cumin
- 1/2 teaspoon smoked paprika
- Salt and pepper to taste
- 1/2 cup shredded low-fat cheese
- Fresh parsley for garnish

Instructions

- Preheat the oven to 375°F (190°C).
- In a bowl, combine cooked quinoa, chopped spinach, black beans, corn, tomato sauce, cumin, smoked paprika, salt, and pepper.
- Spoon the mixture into halved bell peppers.
- Place stuffed peppers in a baking dish.
- Sprinkle shredded cheese over the top.
- Bake the peppers for 25 minutes, or until they become soft.
- Garnish with fresh parsley and serve these tasty DASH Diet Quinoa and Spinach Stuffed Peppers.

Nutritional Facts: 280 calories, 15g protein, 40g carbohydrates, 7g fat, 3g saturated fat, 480mg sodium

34. TUNA SALAD WITH MIXED GREENS

Cooking time: 10 mins   **Yield:** 2

Ingredients

- Two drained 5-ounce cans of tuna each in water
- 4 cups mixed salad greens
- 1 cucumber, sliced
- 1 cup cherry tomatoes, halved
- 1/4 red onion, thinly sliced
- 2 tablespoons olive oil
- 1 tablespoon balsamic vinegar
- 1 teaspoon Dijon mustard
- Salt and pepper to taste
- Lemon wedges for serving

Instructions

- In a bowl, combine drained tuna, mixed salad greens, cucumber, cherry tomatoes, and red onion.
- In a small jar, whisk together olive oil, balsamic vinegar, Dijon mustard, salt, and pepper to create the dressing.
- After drizzling the salad with the dressing, gently toss to coat.
- Serve with lemon wedges and enjoy this refreshing DASH Diet Tuna Salad With Mixed Greens.

Nutritional Facts: 300 calories, 30g protein, 15g carbohydrates, 15g fat, 2.5g saturated fat, 500mg sodium

35.   GRILLED SALMON WITH LEMON DILL DRESSING

Cooking time: 25 min   **Yield:** 10

Ingredients

- 2 salmon fillets
- 1 tablespoon olive oil
- 1 teaspoon lemon zest
- 2 tablespoons lemon juice
- 1 tablespoon fresh dill, chopped
- 1 clove garlic, minced
- Salt and pepper to taste
- Lemon wedges for serving

Instructions

- Preheat the grill to medium-high heat.
- Salmon fillets should be seasoned with salt and pepper and brushed with olive oil.
- Fish should be cooked thoroughly after grilling for 4–5 minutes on each side.
- In a bowl, whisk together lemon zest, lemon juice, chopped dill, minced garlic, salt, and pepper to create the dressing.
- Drizzle the lemon dill dressing over grilled salmon.
- Serve with lemon wedges and enjoy this flavorful DASH Diet Grilled Salmon.

Nutritional Facts: 320 calories, 30g protein, 0g carbohydrates, 20g fat, 3g saturated fat, 400mg sodium

36.   ZUCCHINI NOODLES WITH PESTIS

Cooking time: 20 mins   **Yield:** 4

Ingredients

- 4 medium zucchinis, spiralized
- 1 cup cherry tomatoes, halved
- 1/2 cup pine nuts, toasted
- 1 cup fresh basil leaves
- 1/2 cup grated Parmesan cheese
- 2 cloves garlic
- 1/2 cup olive oil
- Salt and pepper to taste

Instructions

- In a blender or food processor, combine basil, pine nuts, Parmesan, and garlic.
- With the motor running, slowly drizzle in olive oil until the pesto is smooth.
- Season with salt and pepper to taste.
- Sauté zucchini noodles in a big skillet until they are slightly soft.
- Toss zucchini noodles with cherry tomatoes and pesto.
- Serve warm and relish this light and flavorful DASH Diet Zucchini Noodles with Pesto.

Nutritional Facts: 280 calories, 7g protein, 8g carbohydrates, 25g fat, 4g saturated fat, 300mg sodium

Nutritional Facts: 320 calories, 10g protein, 35g carbohydrates, 16g fat, 5g saturated fat, 450mg sodium

37. MEDITERRANEAN QUINOA SALAD

Cooking time: 35 mins   **Yield:** 4

Ingredients

- 1 cup quinoa, cooked and cooled
- 1 cup cucumber, diced
- 1 cup cherry tomatoes, halved
- 1/2 cup Kalamata olives, sliced
- 1/4 cup red onion, finely chopped
- 1/2 cup feta cheese, crumbled
- 2 tablespoons olive oil
- 1 tablespoon red wine vinegar
- 1 teaspoon dried oregano
- Salt and pepper to taste

Instructions

- In a large bowl, combine cooked quinoa, diced cucumber, cherry tomatoes, Kalamata olives, red onion, and crumbled feta cheese.
- Olive oil, red wine vinegar, dried oregano, salt, and pepper should all be combined in a small bowl.
- Over the quinoa mixture, drizzle with the dressing and toss to mix.
- Serve chilled and enjoy the vibrant flavors of this DASH Diet Mediterranean Quinoa Salad.

38. CAPRESE SANDWICH WITH PESTO

Cooking time: 1o mins   **Yield:** 2

Ingredients

- 4 slices whole-grain bread
- 1 large tomato, sliced
- 1 cup fresh mozzarella, sliced
- Fresh basil leaves
- 2 tablespoons homemade or store-bought pesto
- Balsamic glaze for drizzling
- Salt and pepper to taste

Instructions

- On two slices of bread, layer tomato slices, fresh mozzarella, and basil leaves.
- Spread pesto on the remaining two slices of bread.
- Place the pesto-covered slices on top of the tomato-mozzarella-basil layers to form sandwiches.
- Season with Salt and pepper to taste, then drizzle with balsamic glaze.
- Slice and enjoy this light and flavorful DASH Diet Caprese Sandwich with Pesto.

Nutritional Facts: 350 calories, 15g protein, 30g carbohydrates, 18g fat, 7g saturated fat, 450mg sodium

39. PUMPKIN SOUP

Cooking time: 40mins   **Yield:** 4

Ingredients

- 2 cups canned pumpkin puree
- 1 onion, diced
- 2 carrots, peeled and chopped
- 2 cloves garlic, minced
- 4 cups low-sodium vegetable broth
- 1 cup unsweetened almond milk
- 1 teaspoon ground cinnamon
- 1/2 teaspoon ground nutmeg
- Salt and pepper to taste
- Pumpkin seeds for garnish (optional)

Instructions

- In a large pot, sauté diced onion and chopped carrots until softened.
- Add the minced garlic and continue cooking for one more minute.
- Add the vegetable broth, almond milk, ground nutmeg, ground cinnamon, and salt and pepper to the canned pumpkin puree.
- Simmer for twenty to twenty-five minutes, stirring from time to time.
- Blend the soup with an immersion blender until it's smooth.

- If desired, top heated dish with pumpkin seeds.
- Enjoy this comforting and nutritious DASH Diet Pumpkin Soup.

Nutritional Facts: 180 calories, 5g protein, 25g carbohydrates, 8g fat, 1g saturated fat, 400mg sodium

40. BEAN CHILI

Cooking time: 45 mins   **Yield:** 6

Ingredients

- One can (15 oz) of rinsed and drained black beans
- One can (15 oz) of washed and drained kidney beans
- 1 can (15 oz) diced tomatoes
- 1 onion, diced
- 1 bell pepper, diced
- 2 cloves garlic, minced
- 1 cup low-sodium vegetable broth
- 2 tablespoons chili powder
- 1 teaspoon cumin
- Salt and pepper to taste
- Fresh cilantro for garnish

Instructions

- In a large pot, sauté diced onion and bell pepper until softened.
- Add the minced garlic and continue cooking for one more minute..

- Stir in black beans, kidney beans, diced tomatoes, vegetable broth, chili powder, cumin, salt, and pepper.
- Bring to a simmer and let it cook for 25-30 minutes, stirring occasionally.
- Adjust seasoning if needed.
- Serve hot, garnished with fresh cilantro.
- Enjoy this hearty and flavorful DASH Diet Bean Chili.

Nutritional Facts: 250 calories, 12g protein, 45g carbohydrates, 2g fat, 0g saturated fat, 500mg sodium

41.   CAULIFLOWER PIZZA

Cooking time: 45 mins   **Yield:** 4

Ingredients

- 1 medium cauliflower head, grated
- 2 eggs
- 1 cup shredded mozzarella cheese
- 1 teaspoon dried oregano
- 1 teaspoon garlic powder
- Salt and pepper to taste
- 1/2 cup tomato sauce
- 1 cup cherry tomatoes, halved
- 1 cup baby spinach
- 1/4 cup grated Parmesan cheese

Instructions

- Preheat the oven to 400°F (200°C).

- Place grated cauliflower in a clean kitchen towel and squeeze out excess moisture.
- In a bowl, combine cauliflower, eggs, shredded mozzarella, oregano, garlic powder, salt, and pepper to form the pizza crust.
- Press the cauliflower mixture onto a lined baking sheet to form a crust.
- The crust should turn brown after 15 to 20 minutes of baking.
- Spread tomato sauce on the crust, top with cherry tomatoes, baby spinach, and grated Parmesan.
- Bake for a further five to seven minutes, or until the cheese is bubbling and melted.
- Slice and enjoy this delicious and low-carb DASH Diet Cauliflower Pizza.

Nutritional Facts: 200 calories, 12g protein, 15g carbohydrates, 10g fat, 5g saturated fat, 400mg sodium

42.   BAKED MACARONI

Cooking time: 45 mins   **Yield:** 6

Ingredients

- 8 oz whole-grain macaroni
- 2 tablespoons olive oil
- 1 onion, diced
- 2 cloves garlic, minced
- 2 tablespoons whole-grain flour

- 2 cups low-fat milk
- 2 cups shredded sharp cheddar cheese
- 1 teaspoon Dijon mustard
- Salt and pepper to taste
- 1/4 cup breadcrumbs
- Fresh parsley for garnish

Instructions

- Preheat the oven to 375°F (190°C).
- Cook macaroni according to package instructions.
- In a large skillet, sauté diced onion and minced garlic in olive oil until softened.
- Stir in whole-grain flour and cook for 1-2 minutes.
- Gradually whisk in low-fat milk, then add shredded cheddar cheese, Dijon mustard, salt, and pepper.
- Combine the cheese sauce with cooked macaroni and transfer to a baking dish.
- Sprinkle breadcrumbs on top.
- Bake for 20 to 25 minutes, or until bubbling and brown.
- Garnish with fresh parsley and serve this comforting DASH Diet Baked Macaroni.

Nutritional Facts: 350 calories, 18g protein, 35g carbohydrates, 16g fat, 8g saturated fat, 400mg sodium

43. BROWN RICE AND ARUGULA BOWL

Cooking time: 55 mins   **Yield:** 4

Ingredients

- 1 cup brown rice, cooked
- 2 cups arugula
- 1 cup cherry tomatoes, halved
- 1 cucumber, diced
- 1/4 cup feta cheese, crumbled
- 2 tablespoons olive oil
- 1 tablespoon balsamic vinegar
- 1 teaspoon honey
- Salt and pepper to taste
- Pumpkin seeds for garnish (optional)

Instructions

- In a large bowl, combine cooked brown rice, arugula, cherry tomatoes, cucumber, and crumbled feta cheese.
- To make the dressing, combine the olive oil, balsamic vinegar, honey, salt, and pepper in a small bowl.
- Pour the dressing over the rice and vegetable mixture, toss gently to coat.
- Garnish with pumpkin seeds if desired.
- Serve this wholesome and flavorful DASH Diet Brown Rice and Arugula Bowl.

Nutritional Facts: 280 calories, 7g protein, 40g carbohydrates, 10g fat, 3g saturated fat, 300mg sodium

44. CHICKEN RICE

Cooking time: 40 **mins**   **Yield:** 6

Ingredients

- 1 cup brown rice, uncooked
- 1 pound boneless, skinless chicken breasts, diced
- 1 onion, diced
- 2 bell peppers, sliced
- 2 cloves garlic, minced
- 1 cup broccoli florets
- 2 tablespoons olive oil
- 1 teaspoon dried thyme
- 1 teaspoon paprika
- 1/2 teaspoon salt
- 1/4 teaspoon black pepper
- Fresh parsley for garnish

Instructions

- Cook brown rice according to package instructions.
- In a large skillet, sauté diced chicken, diced onion, sliced bell peppers, and minced garlic in olive oil until chicken is cooked through.
- Add broccoli florets and continue cooking for an additional 3-5 minutes.
- Season with dried thyme, paprika, salt, and black pepper.
- Serve the chicken and vegetable mixture over cooked brown rice.
- Garnish with fresh parsley.

- Enjoy this balanced and savory DASH Diet Chicken Rice.

Nutritional Facts: 350 calories, 25g protein, 40g carbohydrates, 10g fat, 2g saturated fat, 400mg sodium

45. VEGETARIAN PITA MEAL

Cooking time: 30 mins   **Yield:** 2

Ingredients

- 2 whole-grain pitas
- 1 cup canned chickpeas, drained and rinsed
- 1 cup cherry tomatoes, halved
- 1 cucumber, diced
- 1/4 cup red onion, thinly sliced
- 1/2 cup feta cheese, crumbled
- 2 tablespoons olive oil
- 1 tablespoon lemon juice
- 1 teaspoon dried oregano
- 1/4 teaspoon salt
- 1/4 teaspoon black pepper
- Fresh mint for garnish

Instructions

- In a bowl, combine chickpeas, cherry tomatoes, diced cucumber, red onion, and crumbled feta cheese.
- In a small jar, whisk together olive oil, lemon juice, dried oregano, salt, and black pepper to create the dressing.

- Toss the salad with the dressing.
- Warm the whole-grain pitas.
- Stuff pitas with the salad mixture.
- Garnish with fresh mint.
- Enjoy this refreshing and nutritious DASH Diet Vegetarian Pita Meal.

Nutritional Facts: 320 calories, 12g protein, 40g carbohydrates, 15g fat, 5g saturated fat, 500mg sodium

46. FLAT BREAD PIZZA

Cooking time: 27 mins   **Yield:** 3

Ingredients

- 3 whole-grain flatbreads
- 1 cup tomato sauce
- 1 cup shredded part-skim mozzarella cheese
- 1 cup cherry tomatoes, halved
- 1/2 cup baby spinach leaves
- 1/4 cup sliced black olives
- 1 teaspoon dried basil
- 1/2 teaspoon dried oregano
- 1/4 teaspoon salt
- 1/4 teaspoon black pepper
- Red pepper flakes for optional heat

Instructions

- Preheat the oven to 400°F (200°C).
- Spread tomato sauce over each flatbread.

- Sprinkle shredded mozzarella evenly on top.
- Arrange cherry tomatoes, baby spinach, and black olives.
- Season with dried basil, dried oregano, salt, black pepper, and optional red pepper flakes.
- Bake the cheese for ten to twelve minutes, or until it is bubbling and melted.
- Slice and relish this flavorful and heart-healthy DASH Diet Flat Bread Pizza.

Nutritional Facts: 280 calories, 12g protein, 40g carbohydrates, 8g fat, 3g saturated fat, 500mg sodium

47. PRAWN STEW

Cooking time: 40 mins   **Yield:** 5

Ingredients

- 1 pound large prawns, peeled and deveined
- 1 onion, diced
- 2 bell peppers, sliced
- 2 cloves garlic, minced
- 1 can (15 oz) diced tomatoes
- 1 cup low-sodium vegetable broth
- 1 teaspoon dried thyme
- 1 teaspoon paprika
- 1/2 teaspoon salt
- 1/4 teaspoon black pepper

- Fresh parsley for garnish

Instructions

- In a large pot, sauté diced onion, sliced bell peppers, and minced garlic until softened.
- Add prawns and cook until they start to turn pink.
- Stir in diced tomatoes, vegetable broth, dried thyme, paprika, salt, and black pepper.
- Bring to a simmer and let it cook for 20-25 minutes, stirring occasionally.
- Adjust seasoning if needed.
- Garnish with fresh parsley.
- Serve this flavorful and protein-packed DASH Diet Prawn Stew.

Nutritional Facts: 220 calories, 25g protein, 15g carbohydrates, 8g fat, 1.5g saturated fat, 400mg sodium

48.   GREEK CHICKEN SALAD

Cooking time: 40 mins   **Yield:** 2

Ingredients

- 2 boneless, skinless chicken breasts
- 4 cups mixed salad greens
- 1 cup cherry tomatoes, halved
- 1 cucumber, sliced
- 1/2 cup Kalamata olives, sliced
- 1/4 cup red onion, thinly sliced
- 1/2 cup feta cheese, crumbled

- 2 tablespoons olive oil
- 1 tablespoon red wine vinegar
- 1 teaspoon dried oregano
- 1/4 teaspoon salt
- 1/4 teaspoon black pepper
- Lemon wedges for serving

Instructions

- Season chicken breasts with salt and pepper.
- Grill or cook chicken until fully cooked.
- In a large bowl, combine mixed salad greens, cherry tomatoes, sliced cucumber, Kalamata olives, red onion, and crumbled feta cheese.
- After grilling, cut the chicken into slices and add it to the salad.
- In a small jar, whisk together olive oil, red wine vinegar, dried oregano, salt, and black pepper to create the dressing.
- Drizzle the dressing over the salad.
- Serve with lemon wedges and enjoy this refreshing DASH Diet Greek Chicken Salad.

Nutritional Facts: 320 calories, 30g protein, 15g carbohydrates, 18g fat, 5g saturated fat, 500mg sodium

49.   TURKEY AND VEGETABLE STIR-FRY

Cooking time: 30 mins   **Yield:** 4

Ingredients

- 1 pound lean ground turkey
- 1 broccoli crown, cut into florets
- 1 bell pepper, sliced
- 1 carrot, julienned
- 1 zucchini, sliced
- 2 tablespoons soy sauce (low-sodium)
- 1 tablespoon hoisin sauce
- 1 teaspoon sesame oil
- 1/2 teaspoon ground ginger
- 1/4 teaspoon salt
- 1/4 teaspoon black pepper
- Green onions for garnish

Instructions

- In a large skillet, brown ground turkey over medium heat.
- Add broccoli florets, sliced bell pepper, julienned carrot, and sliced zucchini. Cook until vegetables are tender-crisp.
- In a small bowl, mix together soy sauce, hoisin sauce, sesame oil, ground ginger, salt, and black pepper.
- Pour the sauce over the turkey and vegetable mixture. Stir to coat evenly.
- Cook for an additional 3-5 minutes.
- Garnish with green onions.
- Serve this protein-rich and colorful DASH Diet Turkey and Vegetable Stir-fry.

Nutritional Facts: 280 calories, 25g protein, 15g carbohydrates, 12g fat, 2.5g saturated fat, 500mg sodium

50.   CHICKEN AND VEGETABLE KABOBS

Cooking time: 25 mins   **Yield:** 1

Ingredients

- One pound of chopped, skinless, and boneless chicken breasts
- 1 bell pepper, cut into squares
- 1 zucchini, sliced
- 1 red onion, cut into wedges
- Cherry tomatoes
- 2 tablespoons olive oil
- 2 tablespoons balsamic vinegar
- 1 teaspoon dried rosemary
- 1/2 teaspoon garlic powder
- 1/4 teaspoon salt
- 1/4 teaspoon black pepper
- Wooden skewers, soaked in water

Instructions

- Turn the heat up to medium-high on the grill or grill pan.
- In a bowl, combine chicken chunks, bell pepper squares, sliced zucchini, red onion wedges, and cherry tomatoes.
- In a small jar, whisk together olive oil, balsamic vinegar, dried rosemary,

garlic powder, salt, and black pepper to create the marinade.

- Pour the marinade over the chicken and vegetables, toss to coat evenly, and let it marinate for at least 15 minutes.
- Thread marinated chicken and vegetables onto soaked wooden skewers.
- Grill the kabobs for about 10-15 minutes, turning occasionally, until the chicken is cooked through and the vegetables are tender.
- Serve these flavorful and colorful DASH Diet Chicken and Vegetable Kabobs.

Nutritional Facts: 280 calories, 25g protein, 15g carbohydrates, 12g fat, 2.5g saturated fat, 400mg sodium

CHAPTER 4

DINNER RECIPES

51. BAKED COD WITH MEDITERRANEAN HERBS

Cooking time: 35 mins   **Yield:** 4

Ingredients

- 4 cod fillets
- 2 tablespoons olive oil
- 1 tablespoon lemon juice
- 2 cloves garlic, minced
- 1 teaspoon dried oregano
- 1 teaspoon dried thyme
- 1/2 teaspoon salt
- 1/4 teaspoon black pepper
- 1/4 teaspoon paprika
- Lemon wedges for serving

Instructions

- Preheat the oven to 400°F (200°C).
- Place cod fillets in a baking dish.
- In a small bowl, whisk together olive oil, lemon juice, minced garlic, dried oregano, dried thyme, salt, black pepper, and paprika.
- Pour the herb mixture over the cod fillets, ensuring they are well-coated.
- Bake the cod for 15 to 20 minutes, or until it's flaky.
- Serve with lemon wedges and savor this light and flavorful DASH Diet Baked Cod.

Nutritional Facts: 220 calories, 30g protein, 1g carbohydrates, 10g fat, 1.5g saturated fat, 400mg sodium

52. BAKED EGGPLANT PARMESAN

Cooking time: 55 mins   **Yield:** 4

Ingredients

- 2 medium-sized eggplants, sliced
- 2 cups tomato sauce (low-sodium)
- 1 cup part-skim mozzarella cheese, shredded
- 1/2 cup Parmesan cheese, grated
- 1/4 cup fresh basil, chopped
- 1 teaspoon dried oregano
- 1/2 teaspoon salt
- 1/4 teaspoon black pepper
- Olive oil cooking spray

Instructions

Preheat the oven to 375°F (190°C).

- Place eggplant slices on a baking sheet, spray with olive oil cooking spray, and bake for 15 minutes, flipping halfway through.

- In a baking dish, layer baked eggplant slices, tomato sauce, mozzarella cheese, Parmesan cheese, chopped fresh basil, dried oregano, salt, and black pepper.
- Until all of the ingredients are utilized, keep layering.
- Bake the cheese for 25 to 30 minutes, or until it is bubbling and melted.
- Allow to cool slightly before serving this hearty and satisfying DASH Diet Baked Eggplant Parmesan..

Nutritional Facts: 280 calories, 15g protein, 25g carbohydrates, 15g fat, 8g saturated fat, 500mg sodium

53.   MEDITERRANEAN COUSCOUS SALAD

Cooking time: 20 mins   **Yield:** 6

Ingredients

- 1 cup whole wheat couscous, cooked and cooled
- 1 cucumber, diced
- 1 cup cherry tomatoes, halved
- 1/2 cup Kalamata olives, spliced
- 1/4 cup red onion, finely chopped
- 1/2 cup feta cheese, crumbled
- 2 tablespoons olive oil
- 1 tablespoon red wine vinegar
- 1 teaspoon dried oregano
- 1/4 teaspoon salt
- 1/4 teaspoon black pepper
- Fresh parsley for garnish

Instructions

- In a large bowl, combine cooked and cooled whole wheat couscous, diced cucumber, cherry tomatoes, sliced Kalamata olives, chopped red onion, and crumbled feta cheese.
- In a small bowl, whisk together olive oil, red wine vinegar, dried oregano, salt, and black pepper to create the dressing.
- Pour the dressing over the couscous mixture and toss gently to coat.
- Garnish with fresh parsley and serve this vibrant and wholesome DASH Diet Mediterranean Couscous Salad.

Nutritional Facts: 220 calories, 7g protein, 35g carbohydrates, 8g fat, 3g saturated fat, 400mg sodium

54.   LEMON GARLIC CHICKEN WITH ASPARAGUS

Cooking time: 40 mins   **Yield:** 4

Ingredients

- 4 boneless, skinless chicken breasts
- 1 bunch asparagus, trimmed
- 3 tablespoons olive oil

- 3 cloves garlic, minced
- Zest and juice of 1 lemon
- 1 teaspoon dried thyme
- 1/2 teaspoon salt
- 1/4 teaspoon black pepper
- Fresh parsley for garnish

Instructions

- Preheat the oven to 400°F (200°C).
- Place chicken breasts and trimmed asparagus on a baking sheet.
- In a bowl, whisk together olive oil, minced garlic, lemon zest, lemon juice, dried thyme, salt, and black pepper.
- Pour the mixture over the chicken and asparagus, ensuring they are well-coated.
- Bake for 20-25 minutes or until the chicken is cooked through and the asparagus is tender.
- Garnish with fresh parsley and savor this light and flavorful DASH Diet Lemon Garlic Chicken.

Nutritional Facts: 280 calories, 30g protein, 7g carbohydrates, 15g fat, 2.5g saturated fat, 400mg sodium

- 4 salmon fillets
- 3 tablespoons Dijon mustard
- 2 tablespoons honey
- 1 tablespoon olive oil
- 1 teaspoon soy sauce (low-sodium)
- 1/2 teaspoon dried rosemary
- 1/4 teaspoon salt
- 1/4 teaspoon black pepper
- Lemon wedges for serving

Instructions

- Preheat the oven to 400°F (200°C).
- In a small bowl, mix together Dijon mustard, honey, olive oil, soy sauce, dried rosemary, salt, and black pepper.
- Place salmon fillets on a baking sheet and brush them with the honey mustard mixture.
- Bake the salmon for 12 to 15 minutes, or until it is tender.
- Serve with lemon wedges and relish this sweet and savory DASH Diet Honey Mustard Glazed Salmon.

Nutritional Facts: 300 calories, 25g protein, 10g carbohydrates, 18g fat, 3g saturated fat, 400mg sodium

55. HONEY MUSTARD GLAZED SALMON

Cooking time: 25 mins　　　**Yield:** 4

Ingredients

56. LEMON HERB QUINOA WITH GRILLED CHICKEN

Cooking time: 35 mins　　　**Yield:** 4

Ingredients

- 1 cup quinoa, cooked
- 4 boneless, skinless chicken breasts
- 2 tablespoons olive oil
- Zest and juice of 1 lemon
- 2 tablespoons fresh herbs (such as parsley, basil, or chives), chopped
- 1/2 teaspoon dried oregano
- 1/4 teaspoon salt
- 1/4 teaspoon black pepper
- Cherry tomatoes for garnish

Instructions

- Cook quinoa according to package instructions.
- Season chicken breasts with olive oil, lemon zest, lemon juice, fresh herbs, dried oregano, salt, and black pepper.
- Grill chicken until fully cooked.
- Fluff the cooked quinoa with a fork and serve topped with grilled chicken.
- Garnish with cherry tomatoes.
- Enjoy this wholesome and satisfying DASH Diet Lemon Herb Quinoa With Grilled Chicken.

Nutritional Facts: 320 calories, 30g protein, 20g carbohydrates, 15g fat, 2.5g saturated fat, 400mg sodium

57.   CHICKPEA AND SPINACH STEW

Cooking time: 40 mins   **Yield:** 4

Ingredients

- Two cans (15 oz each) of rinsed and drained chickpeas
- 1 onion, diced
- 2 cloves garlic, minced
- 1 can (14 oz) diced tomatoes
- 1 teaspoon ground cumin
- 1 teaspoon smoked paprika
- 1/2 teaspoon ground coriander
- 1/2 teaspoon salt
- 1/4 teaspoon black pepper
- 4 cups fresh spinach
- 1 lemon, juiced
- Olive oil for drizzling

Instructions

- In a large pot, sauté diced onion and minced garlic until softened.
- Add chickpeas, diced tomatoes, ground cumin, smoked paprika, ground coriander, salt, and black pepper.
- Bring to a simmer and cook for 20-25 minutes.
- Add fresh spinach and lemon juice, stir until the spinach is wilted.
- Drizzle with olive oil before serving this protein-packed and flavorful DASH Diet Chickpea and Spinach Stew.

Nutritional Facts: 250 calories, 12g protein, 40g carbohydrates, 5g fat, 0.5g saturated fat, 500mg sodium

58.   MEXICAN QUINOA SKILLET

Cooking time: 35 mins   **Yield:** 4

Ingredients

- 1 cup quinoa, uncooked
- 1 pound lean ground turkey
- 1 onion, diced
- 1 bell pepper, diced
- A fifteen-ounce can of drained and rinsed black beans
- 1 cup corn kernels
- One can of chopped tomatoes with green chiles, 14 ounces
- 1 teaspoon chili powder
- 1/2 teaspoon cumin
- 1/2 teaspoon salt
- 1/4 teaspoon black pepper
- Fresh cilantro for garnish

Instructions

- Cook quinoa according to package instructions.
- In a large skillet, brown ground turkey with diced onion and bell pepper.
- Add black beans, corn kernels, diced tomatoes with green chilies, chili powder, cumin, salt, and black pepper.
- Stir in cooked quinoa and simmer for 5-7 minutes.
- Garnish with fresh cilantro before serving this protein-rich and satisfying DASH Diet Mexican Quinoa Skillet.

Nutritional Facts: 320 calories, 25g protein, 40g carbohydrates, 8g fat, 2g saturated fat, 500mg sodium

59.   CAPRESE STUFFED CHICKEN BREAST

Cooking time: 40 mins   **Yield:** 4

Ingredients

- 4 boneless, skinless chicken breasts
- 1 cup cherry tomatoes, halved
- 1 cup fresh mozzarella, diced
- 1/4 cup fresh basil, chopped
- 2 tablespoons balsamic glaze
- 1 teaspoon dried oregano
- 1/2 teaspoon salt
- 1/4 teaspoon black pepper
- Olive oil for drizzling

Instructions

- Preheat the oven to 400°F (200°C).
- Slice a pocket into each chicken breast.
- In a bowl, mix cherry tomatoes, fresh mozzarella, chopped fresh basil, balsamic glaze, dried oregano, salt, and black pepper.
- Stuff each chicken breast with the caprese mixture.

- Drizzle with olive oil and bake for 20-25 minutes or until the chicken is cooked through.
- Serve this elegant and delicious DASH Diet Caprese Stuffed Chicken Breast.

Nutritional Facts: 280 calories, 30g protein, 5g carbohydrates, 15g fat, 6g saturated fat, 500mg sodium

60. RATATOUILLE WITH WHOLE WHEAT COUSCOUS

Cooking time: 50 mins   **Yield:** 4

Ingredients

- 1 eggplant, diced
- 2 zucchinis, sliced
- 1 bell pepper, diced
- 1 onion, diced
- 2 cloves garlic, minced
- 1 can (14 oz) diced tomatoes
- 2 tablespoons tomato paste
- 1 teaspoon dried thyme
- 1 teaspoon dried rosemary
- 1/2 teaspoon salt
- 1/4 teaspoon black pepper
- 1 cup whole wheat couscous, cooked
- Fresh basil for garnish

Instructions

- In a large pot, sauté diced onion and minced garlic until softened.

- Add diced eggplant, sliced zucchini, diced bell pepper, diced tomatoes, tomato paste, dried thyme, dried rosemary, salt, and black pepper.
- Simmer for 25-30 minutes until vegetables are tender.
- Serve over cooked whole wheat couscous and garnish with fresh basil for a hearty and flavorful DASH Diet Ratatouille.

Nutritional Facts: 280 calories, 7g protein, 55g carbohydrates, 3g fat, 0.5g saturated fat, 500mg sodium

61. ITALIAN HERB GRILLED PORK CHOPS

Cooking time: 55 mins   **Yield:** 4

Ingredients

- 4 bone-in pork chops
- 2 tablespoons olive oil
- 1 tablespoon balsamic vinegar
- 1 teaspoon dried oregano
- 1 teaspoon dried basil
- 1/2 teaspoon garlic powder
- 1/2 teaspoon salt
- 1/4 teaspoon black pepper

Instructions

- In a bowl, mix the olive oil, balsamic vinegar, dried oregano, dried basil, garlic powder, salt, and black pepper together.

- Marinate pork chops in the mixture for at least 30 minutes.
- Preheat the grill to medium-high heat.
- Grill pork chops for 6-8 minutes per side or until fully cooked.
- Allow to rest for a few minutes before serving these flavorful and lean DASH Diet Italian Herb Grilled Pork Chops.

Nutritional Facts: 280 calories, 30g protein, 1g carbohydrates, 18g fat, 5g saturated fat, 500mg sodium

62. SPICY SHRIMP STIR-FRY WITH BROWN RICE

Cooking time: 25 mins   **Yield:** 4

Ingredients

- 1 pound large shrimp, peeled and deveined
- 2 cups broccoli florets
- 1 red bell pepper, sliced
- 1 carrot, julienned
- 2 tablespoons soy sauce (low-sodium)
- 1 tablespoon sriracha
- 1 tablespoon sesame oil
- 1 teaspoon ginger, minced
- 1/2 teaspoon salt
- 1/4 teaspoon black pepper
- 2 cups cooked brown rice

Instructions

- Sesame oil should be heated over medium-high heat in a wok or big skillet.
- Add shrimp and stir-fry until pink, then add broccoli, sliced red bell pepper, and julienned carrot.
- In a small bowl, mix the soy sauce, sriracha, minced ginger, salt, and black pepper together.
- Pour the sauce over the shrimp and vegetables, and stir-fry for an additional 3-5 minutes.
- Serve over cooked brown rice for a spicy and protein-packed DASH Diet Spicy Shrimp Stir-fry.

Nutritional Facts: 320 calories, 25g protein, 40g carbohydrates, 8g fat, 1.5g saturated fat, 600mg sodium

63. SPICY SHRIMP, VEGETABLE & COUSCOUS BOWLS

Cooking time: 35mins   **Yield:** 4

Ingredients

- 1 pound large shrimp, peeled and deveined
- Two cups of mixed veggies, including cherry tomatoes, zucchini, and bell peppers
- 1 cup whole wheat couscous, cooked

- 2 tablespoons olive oil
- 1 tablespoon harissa paste
- 1 teaspoon smoked paprika
- 1/2 teaspoon cumin
- 1/2 teaspoon salt
- 1/4 teaspoon black pepper
- Fresh cilantro for garnish

Instructions

- Preheat the oven to 400°F (200°C).
- In a bowl, toss shrimp and mixed vegetables with olive oil, harissa paste, smoked paprika, cumin, salt, and black pepper.
- Spread the mixture on a baking sheet and roast for 12-15 minutes.
- Serve over cooked whole wheat couscous, garnished with fresh cilantro for a flavorful and nutritious DASH Diet Spicy Shrimp Bowl..

Nutritional Facts: 320 calories, 25g protein, 40g carbohydrates, 8g fat, 1.5g saturated fat, 600mg sodium

64. SHEET-PAN HARISSA CHICKEN & VEGETABLES

Cooking time: 70 mins   **Yield:** 4

Ingredients

- 4 boneless, skinless chicken breasts
- 1 cup baby potatoes, halved
- 1 cup baby carrots

- 1 cup broccoli florets
- 2 tablespoons olive oil
- 2 tablespoons harissa paste
- 1 teaspoon cumin
- 1 teaspoon paprika
- 1/2 teaspoon salt
- 1/4 teaspoon black pepper
- Lemon wedges for serving

Instructions

- In a bowl, mix together olive oil, harissa paste, cumin, paprika, salt, and black pepper.
- Give the chicken breasts at least 30 minutes to marinate in the marinade.
- Preheat the oven to 400°F (200°C).
- Place marinated chicken breasts, halved baby potatoes, baby carrots, and broccoli florets on a baking sheet.
- Roast for 25 minutes or until the chicken is cooked through and vegetables are tender.
- Serve with lemon wedges for a zesty DASH Diet Sheet-Pan Harissa Chicken & Vegetables.

Nutritional Facts: 300 calories, 30g protein, 25g carbohydrates, 10g fat, 1.5g saturated fat, 600mg sodium

65. WALNUT-ROSEMARY CRUSTED SALMON

Cooking time: 30 mins   **Yield:** 2

Ingredients

- 4 salmon fillets
- 1/2 cup walnuts, finely chopped
- 2 tablespoons fresh rosemary, chopped
- 2 tablespoons Dijon mustard
- 1 tablespoon olive oil
- 1 teaspoon lemon zest
- 1/2 teaspoon salt
- 1/4 teaspoon black pepper

Instructions

- Preheat the oven to 400°F (200°C).
- In a bowl, mix together chopped walnuts, fresh rosemary, Dijon mustard, olive oil, lemon zest, salt, and black pepper.
- Place salmon fillets on a baking sheet and press the walnut-rosemary mixture onto the top of each fillet.
- Bake for 12-15 minutes or until the salmon is flaky and the crust is golden.
- Serve this omega-3-rich and flavorful DASH Diet Walnut-Rosemary Crusted Salmon.

Nutritional Facts: 320 calories, 30g protein, 5g carbohydrates, 20g fat, 2.5g saturated fat, 600mg sodium

Ingredients

- 1 pound large shrimp, peeled and deveined
- 8 oz whole wheat linguine, uncooked
- 4 cups fresh spinach
- 4 cloves garlic, minced
- 2 tablespoons olive oil
- 1 teaspoon red pepper flakes
- 1/2 teaspoon salt
- 1/4 teaspoon black pepper
- Lemon wedges for serving

Instructions

- Cook whole wheat linguine according to package instructions.
- Minced garlic should be cooked in olive oil in a big pot until aromatic.
- Add shrimp, fresh spinach, red pepper flakes, salt, and black pepper. Cook until shrimp are pink and spinach is wilted.
- Toss in cooked linguine, ensuring everything is well-coated.
- Serve with lemon wedges for a zesty and nutritious DASH Diet Garlicky Shrimp & Spinach.

Nutritional Facts: 350 calories, 25g protein, 45g carbohydrates, 10g fat, 1.5g saturated fat, 600mg sodium

66. ONE-POT GARLICKY SHRIMP & SPINACH

Cooking time: 30 mins   **Yield:** 4

67. ROASTED SALMON WITH SMOKY CHICKPEAS & GREENS

Cooking time: 45 mins   **Yield:** 4

Ingredients

- 4 salmon filets
- One can (15 oz) of rinsed and drained chickpeas
- 4 cups mixed greens (kale, arugula, spinach)
- 2 tablespoons smoked paprika
- 1 tablespoon olive oil
- 1 teaspoon cumin
- 1/2 teaspoon salt
- 1/4 teaspoon black pepper
- Lemon wedges for serving

Instructions

- Preheat the oven to 400°F (200°C).
- In a bowl, toss chickpeas with smoked paprika, olive oil, cumin, salt, and black pepper.
- Place salmon fillets and chickpeas on a baking sheet.
- Roast for 20-25 minutes or until the salmon is flaky and the chickpeas are crispy.
- Serve over mixed greens with lemon wedges for a protein-packed and smoky DASH Diet Salmon.

Nutritional Facts: 320 calories, 30g protein, 25g carbohydrates, 15g fat, 2.5g saturated fat, 600mg sodium

68. BEEF & BEAN SLOPPY JOES

Cooking time: 35 mins   **Yield:** 4

Ingredients

- 1 pound lean ground beef
- One can (15 oz) of washed and drained kidney beans
- 1 onion, diced
- 1 bell pepper, diced
- 1 cup tomato sauce (low-sodium)
- 2 tablespoons tomato paste
- 1 tablespoon Worcestershire sauce
- 1 teaspoon chili powder
- 1/2 teaspoon salt
- 1/4 teaspoon black pepper
- Whole wheat burger buns for serving

Instructions

- In a skillet, brown ground beef with diced onion and bell pepper.
- Add kidney beans, tomato sauce, tomato paste, Worcestershire sauce, chili powder, salt, and black pepper. Simmer for 15 minutes.
- Serve the flavorful beef and bean mixture on whole wheat burger buns for a satisfying and balanced DASH Diet Sloppy Joe.

Nutritional Facts: 300 calories, 25g protein, 30g carbohydrates, 10g fat, 3.5g saturated fat, 600mg sodium

69. SHEET-PAN CHILI-LIME SALMON WITH POTATOES & PEPPERS

Cooking time: 45 mins   **Yield:** 4

Ingredients

- 4 salmon fillets
- 1 pound baby potatoes, halved
- 2 bell peppers, sliced
- 2 tablespoons olive oil
- Zest and juice of 2 limes
- 1 teaspoon chili powder
- 1/2 teaspoon cumin
- 1/2 teaspoon salt
- 1/4 teaspoon black pepper
- Fresh cilantro for garnish

Instructions

- Preheat the oven to 400°F (200°C).
- Place salmon fillets, halved baby potatoes, and sliced bell peppers on a baking sheet.
- In a bowl, mix together olive oil, lime zest, lime juice, chili powder, cumin, salt, and black pepper.
- Drizzle the mixture over the ingredients on the baking sheet and toss to coat.

- Roast for 20-25 minutes or until salmon is flaky and vegetables are tender.
- Garnish with fresh cilantro for a zesty and nutritious DASH Diet Chili-Lime Salmon.

Nutritional Facts: 320 calories, 30g protein, 25g carbohydrates, 15g fat, 2.5g saturated fat, 600mg sodium

70. SWEET POTATO WEDGES AND BRUSSELS SPROUTS WITH MAPLE-ROASTED CHICKEN THINGS

Cooking time: 80 mins   **Yield:** 4

Ingredients

- 4 bone-in, skin-on chicken thighs
- 2 sweet potatoes, cut into wedges
- 1 pound Brussels sprouts, trimmed and halved
- 3 tablespoons maple syrup
- 2 tablespoons olive oil
- 1 teaspoon dried thyme
- 1/2 teaspoon salt
- 1/4 teaspoon black pepper
- Pecans for garnish

Instructions

- In a bowl, mix together maple syrup, olive oil, dried thyme, salt, and black pepper.

- Marinate chicken thighs, sweet potato wedges, and Brussels sprouts in the mixture for at least 30 minutes.
- Preheat the oven to 425°F (220°C).
- Place marinated ingredients on a baking sheet and roast for 30 minutes or until chicken is cooked through and vegetables are caramelized.
- Garnish with pecans for a sweet and savory DASH Diet Maple-Roasted Chicken Thighs.

Nutritional Facts: 350 calories, 25g protein, 35g carbohydrates, 15g fat, 3.5g saturated fat, 600mg sodium

71.   ONE-PAN CHICKEN & ASPARAGUS BAKE

Cooking time: 40 mins   **Yield:** 4

Ingredients

- 4 boneless, skinless chicken breasts
- 1 pound asparagus, trimmed
- 1 cup cherry tomatoes, halved
- 3 tablespoons balsamic vinegar
- 2 tablespoons olive oil
- 1 teaspoon dried rosemary
- 1/2 teaspoon salt
- 1/4 teaspoon black pepper
- Fresh basil for garnish

Instructions

- Preheat the oven to 400°F (200°C).

- Place chicken breasts, trimmed asparagus, and halved cherry tomatoes in a baking dish.
- In a bowl, whisk together balsamic vinegar, olive oil, dried rosemary, salt, and black pepper.
- Pour the mixture over the ingredients in the baking dish and toss to coat.
- Bake the chicken for 20 to 25 minutes, or until it is thoroughly done.
- Garnish with fresh basil for a simple and delightful DASH Diet Chicken & Asparagus Bake.

Nutritional Facts: 280 calories, 30g protein, 15g carbohydrates, 12g fat, 2.5g saturated fat, 600mg sodium

72.   LENTIL STEW WITH SALSA VERDE

Cooking time: 35 mins   **Yield:** 6

Ingredients

- 1 cup dried green lentils, rinsed
- 1 onion, diced
- 2 carrots, diced
- 2 celery stalks, diced
- 4 cups vegetable broth (low-sodium)
- 1 can (14 oz) diced tomatoes
- 2 cloves garlic, minced
- 2 teaspoons cumin
- 1 teaspoon smoked paprika
- 1/2 teaspoon salt

- 1/4 teaspoon black pepper
- Salsa verde for topping

Instructions

- In a pot, sauté diced onion, carrots, and celery until softened.
- Add dried lentils, vegetable broth, diced tomatoes, minced garlic, cumin, smoked paprika, salt, and black pepper.
- Bring to a boil, then reduce heat and simmer for 30-40 minutes until lentils are tender.
- Serve with a dollop of salsa verde for a flavorful and protein-rich DASH Diet Lentil Stew.

Nutritional Facts: 280 calories, 18g protein, 50g carbohydrates, 2g fat, 0.5g saturated fat, 600mg sodium

73. CHICKPEA PASTA WITH MUSHROOMS & KALE

Cooking time: 55 mins   **Yield:** 4

Ingredients

- 8 oz chickpea pasta
- 2 cups kale, chopped
- 1 cup mushrooms, sliced
- 2 tablespoons olive oil
- 2 cloves garlic, minced
- 1/2 teaspoon red pepper flakes
- 1/2 teaspoon salt

- 1/4 teaspoon black pepper
- Grated Parmesan for topping

Instructions

- Cook chickpea pasta according to package instructions.
- In a skillet, sauté chopped kale and sliced mushrooms in olive oil until softened.
- Add minced garlic, red pepper flakes, salt, and black pepper.
- Toss cooked pasta with the vegetable mixture and top with grated Parmesan for a fiber-rich DASH Diet Chickpea Pasta.

Nutritional Facts: 320 calories, 15g protein, 45g carbohydrates, 10g fat, 1.5g saturated fat, 500mg sodium

74. SPICE-SEARED SALMON WITH GREEK-STYLE GREEN BEANS

Cooking time: 30 mins   **Yield:** 4

Ingredients

- 4 salmon fillets
- 1 pound green beans, trimmed
- 1 cup cherry tomatoes, halved
- 1/4 cup Kalamata olives, sliced
- 2 tablespoons olive oil
- 1 teaspoon dried oregano
- 1/2 teaspoon salt

- 1/4 teaspoon black pepper
- Lemon wedges for serving

Instructions

- Season salmon fillets with dried oregano, salt, and black pepper.
- In a skillet, sear salmon fillets in olive oil until golden on each side.
- Remove salmon from the skillet and add trimmed green beans, halved cherry tomatoes, and sliced Kalamata olives.
- Sauté until vegetables are tender and slightly charred.
- Serve salmon over Greek-style green beans with lemon wedges for an omega-3-rich and flavorful DASH Diet dish.

Nutritional Facts: 320 calories, 25g protein, 15g carbohydrates, 18g fat, 2.5g saturated fat, 600mg sodium

75. LEMON-HERB SALMON WITH CAPONATA & FARRO

Cooking time: 70 mins   **Yield:** 4

Ingredients

- 4 salmon filets
- 1 cup farro, cooked
- 1 eggplant, diced
- 1 zucchini, diced
- 1 bell pepper, diced

- 1 cup cherry tomatoes, halved
- 1/4 cup Kalamata olives, sliced
- 2 tablespoons olive oil
- 2 tablespoons lemon juice
- 1 tablespoon fresh parsley, chopped
- 1 teaspoon dried thyme
- 1/2 teaspoon salt
- 1/4 teaspoon black pepper

Instructions

- Preheat the oven to 400°F (200°C).
- Season salmon fillets with dried thyme, salt, and black pepper.
- In a bowl, toss diced eggplant, zucchini, bell pepper, cherry tomatoes, and sliced Kalamata olives with olive oil.
- Spread the vegetable mixture on a baking sheet and place seasoned salmon fillets on top.
- Drizzle lemon juice over the salmon and vegetables.
- Bake for 20-25 minutes or until salmon is flaky and vegetables are tender.
- Serve the lemon-herb salmon over a bed of cooked farro, garnished with fresh parsley for a delightful DASH Diet meal.

Nutritional Facts: 350 calories, 30g protein, 30g carbohydrates, 15g fat, 2.5g saturated fat, 600mg sodium

CHAPTER 5

MEAT & POULTRY RECIPES

76.   BEEF AND SWEET POTATO HASH

Cooking time: 40 mins   **Yield**: 4

Ingredients

- 1 pound lean ground beef
- 2 sweet potatoes, diced
- 1 onion, diced
- 1 bell pepper, diced
- 2 tablespoons olive oil
- 1 teaspoon smoked paprika
- 1/2 teaspoon cumin
- 1/2 teaspoon salt
- 1/4 teaspoon black pepper
- Fresh cilantro for garnish

Instructions

- In a skillet, brown ground beef with diced onion and bell pepper in olive oil.
- Add diced sweet potatoes, smoked paprika, cumin, salt, and black pepper. Cook until sweet potatoes are tender.
- Serve the flavorful beef and sweet potato hash, garnished with fresh cilantro for a hearty DASH Diet meal.

Nutritional Facts: 320 calories, 25g protein, 30g carbohydrates, 12g fat, 3g saturated fat, 600mg sodium

77.   BEEF AND VEGETABLE CURRY WITH BROWN RICE

Cooking time: 59 mins   **Yield:** 4

Ingredients

- 1 pound lean stew beef, cubed
- 2 cups mixed vegetables (carrots, peas, bell peppers)
- 1 onion, chopped
- 2 cloves garlic, minced
- 1 can (14 oz) diced tomatoes
- 1/2 cup coconut milk (unsweetened)
- 2 tablespoons curry powder
- 1 tablespoon olive oil
- 1/2 teaspoon salt
- 1/4 teaspoon black pepper
- Cooked brown rice for serving

Instructions

- In a pot, sauté chopped onion and minced garlic in olive oil until softened.

- Add cubed stew beef and brown on all sides.
- Stir in mixed vegetables, diced tomatoes, coconut milk, curry powder, salt, and black pepper.
- Simmer until the beef is tender and the curry has thickened.
- Serve over cooked brown rice for a rich and aromatic DASH Diet Beef and Vegetable Curry.

Nutritional Facts: 350 calories, 30g protein, 35g carbohydrates, 12g fat, 4g saturated fat, 600mg sodium

78.   BEEF AND VEGETABLE SOUP WITH WHOLE WHEAT BREAD

Cooking time: 55 mins   **Yield:** 6

Ingredients

- 1 pound lean ground beef
- 2 carrots, sliced
- 2 celery stalks, sliced
- 1 onion, diced
- 2 cloves garlic, minced
- 4 cups low-sodium beef broth
- 1 can (14 oz) diced tomatoes
- 1 cup green beans, chopped
- 1 teaspoon dried thyme
- 1/2 teaspoon salt
- 1/4 teaspoon black pepper
- Whole wheat bread for serving

Instructions

- In a pot, brown ground beef with diced onion and minced garlic.
- Add sliced carrots, celery, diced tomatoes, chopped green beans, dried thyme, salt, and black pepper.
- Pour in low-sodium beef broth and simmer until vegetables are tender.
- Serve the hearty beef and vegetable soup with slices of whole wheat bread for a comforting DASH Diet meal.

Nutritional Facts: Calories 269kcal, Fat 18g, Carbohydrates 6g, Protein 21g, Sodium 350mg, Calcium 27mg. Phosphorus 139mg, Potassium 286mg

79.   HONEY MUSTARD TURKEY BREASTY

Cooking time: 1 hr 40 mins   **Yield:** 6

Ingredients

- 1.5 pounds turkey breast, boneless and skinless
- 1/4 cup Dijon mustard
- 2 tablespoons honey
- 1 tablespoon olive oil
- 1 tablespoon apple cider vinegar
- 1 teaspoon dried thyme
- 1/2 teaspoon salt
- 1/4 teaspoon black pepper

Instructions

- In a bowl, whisk together Dijon mustard, honey, olive oil, apple cider vinegar, dried thyme, salt, and black pepper.
- Marinate turkey breast in the mixture for at least 1 hour.
- Preheat the oven to 375°F (190°C).
- Roast turkey breast for 30 minutes or until cooked through.
- Slice and serve the honey mustard turkey breast for a sweet and savory DASH Diet meal.

Nutritional Facts: Calories 279kcal, Fat 6g, Carbohydrates 38g, Protein 17g, Sodium 196mg, Calcium 52mg. Phosphorus 180mg, Potassium 349mg

80. GRILLED LEMON PEPPER TURKEY BREAST

Cooking time: 2hr 30 mins   **Yield:** 6

Ingredients

- 1.5 pounds turkey breast, boneless and skinless
- Juice and zest of 2 lemons
- 2 tablespoons olive oil
- 1 teaspoon black pepper
- 1 teaspoon dried rosemary
- 1/2 teaspoon salt
- 1/4 teaspoon garlic powder

Instructions

- In a bowl, mix together lemon juice, lemon zest, olive oil, black pepper, dried rosemary, salt, and garlic powder.
- Marinate turkey breast in the mixture for at least 2 hours.
- Preheat the grill to medium-high heat.
- Grill turkey breast for 15-20 minutes, turning occasionally, until cooked through.
- Let it rest for a few minutes before slicing and serving the grilled lemon pepper turkey breast.

Nutritional Facts: 280 calories, 30g protein, 5g carbohydrates, 15g fat, 2.5g saturated fat, 600mg sodium

81. CHICKEN AND VEGETABLE SKEWERS WITH PEANUT SAUCE

Cooking time: 1 hr 35 mins   **Yield:** 4

Ingredients

- 1 pound chicken breast, cut into cubes
- 2 bell peppers, cut into chunks
- 1 zucchini, sliced
- 1/2 cup low-sodium soy sauce
- 2 tablespoons peanut butter

- 1 tablespoon honey
- 1 tablespoon sesame oil
- 1 teaspoon ginger, grated
- 1/2 teaspoon salt
- 1/4 teaspoon black pepper

Instructions

- In a bowl, whisk together low-sodium soy sauce, peanut butter, honey, sesame oil, grated ginger, salt, and black pepper.
- Marinate chicken cubes, bell pepper chunks, and zucchini slices in the mixture for at least 1 hour.
- Preheat the grill to medium-high heat.
- Thread marinated chicken and vegetables onto skewers.
- Grill skewers for 10-15 minutes, turning occasionally, until chicken is cooked and vegetables are tender.
- Serve the chicken and vegetable skewers with peanut sauce for a flavorful DASH Diet dish.

Nutritional Facts: 320 calories, 25g protein, 20g carbohydrates, 15g fat, 3g saturated fat, 600mg sodium

82. GRILLED CHILI LIME CHICKEN

Cooking time: 2 hr 35 mins   **Yield:** 4

Ingredients

- 1.5 pounds chicken breasts
- Zest and juice of 2 limes
- 2 tablespoons olive oil
- 1 tablespoon chili powder
- 1 teaspoon cumin
- 1/2 teaspoon salt
- 1/4 teaspoon black pepper

Instructions

- In a bowl, combine lime zest, lime juice, olive oil, chili powder, cumin, salt, and black pepper.
- Marinate chicken breasts in the mixture for at least 2 hours.
- Preheat the grill to medium-high heat.
- Grill chicken for 15-20 minutes, turning occasionally, until fully cooked.
- Slice and serve the flavorful grilled chili lime chicken for a zesty DASH Diet meal.

Nutritional Facts: 280 calories, 30g protein, 3g carbohydrates, 15g fat, 2.5g saturated fat, 600mg sodium

83. ROSEMARY DIJON CHICKEN

Cooking time: 1 hr 40 mins   **Yield:** 4

Ingredients

- 1.5 pounds chicken thighs, bone-in and skin-on
- 2 tablespoons Dijon mustard
- 2 tablespoons olive oil
- 1 tablespoon fresh rosemary, chopped
- 1 teaspoon garlic powder
- 1/2 teaspoon salt
- 1/4 teaspoon black pepper

Instructions

- In a bowl, mix Dijon mustard, olive oil, chopped rosemary, garlic powder, salt, and black pepper.
- Marinate chicken thighs in the mixture for at least 1 hour.
- Preheat the oven to 400°F (200°C).
- Roast chicken thighs for 25 minutes or until golden and cooked through.
- Serve the rosemary Dijon chicken thighs for a herby and satisfying DASH Diet meal.

Nutritional Facts: 320 calories, 25g protein, 1g carbohydrates, 22g fat, 5g saturated fat, 600mg sodium

84. CILANTRO LIME CHICKEN TENDERS

Cooking time: 1hr 5mins   **Yield:** 4

Ingredients

- 1 pound chicken tenders
- Zest and juice of 1 lime
- 1/4 cup fresh cilantro, chopped
- 2 tablespoons olive oil
- 1 teaspoon cumin
- 1/2 teaspoon paprika
- 1/2 teaspoon salt
- 1/4 teaspoon black pepper

Instructions

- In a bowl, combine lime zest, lime juice, chopped cilantro, olive oil, cumin, paprika, salt, and black pepper.
- Marinate chicken tenders in the mixture for 30 minutes.
- Preheat the oven to 375°F (190°C).
- Bake chicken tenders for 15 minutes or until cooked through.
- Serve the cilantro lime chicken tenders for a fresh and flavorful DASH Diet meal.

Nutritional Facts: 250 calories, 30g protein, 2g carbohydrates, 12g fat, 2g saturated fat, 600mg sodium

85. TOMATO BASIL CHICKEN

Cooking time: 40 mins   **Yield:** 8

Ingredients

- 1.5 pounds chicken breasts
- 2 cups cherry tomatoes, halved

- 1/4 cup fresh basil, chopped
- 2 tablespoons olive oil
- 2 cloves garlic, minced
- 1 teaspoon balsamic vinegar
- 1/2 teaspoon salt
- 1/4 teaspoon black pepper

Instructions

- Salt and black pepper are used to season chicken breasts.
- In a skillet, heat olive oil and sauté chicken until golden brown and cooked through.
- Add minced garlic, cherry tomatoes, chopped basil, and balsamic vinegar.
- Cook for an additional 5 minutes until tomatoes are softened.
- Serve the tomato basil chicken for a light and flavorful DASH Diet meal.

Nutritional Facts: 280 calories, 30g protein, 6g carbohydrates, 14g fat, 2.5g saturated fat, 600mg sodium

86. BEEF AND SPINACH SALAD

Cooking time: 23 mins   **Yield:** 4

Ingredients

- 1 pound lean beef sirloin, sliced
- 6 cups fresh spinach

- 1 cup cherry tomatoes, halved
- 1/2 cup red onion, thinly sliced
- 1/4 cup feta cheese, crumbled
- 2 tablespoons olive oil
- 1 tablespoon balsamic vinegar
- 1 teaspoon Dijon mustard
- 1/2 teaspoon salt
- 1/4 teaspoon black pepper

Instructions

- In a skillet, cook sliced beef until browned.
- In a large bowl, combine fresh spinach, cherry tomatoes, sliced red onion, and crumbled feta cheese.
- Whisk together olive oil, balsamic vinegar, Dijon mustard, salt, and black pepper to make the dressing.
- Toss the cooked beef with the salad and drizzle with the dressing.
- Serve the beef and spinach salad for a protein-packed DASH Diet meal.

Nutritional Facts: 320 calories, 25g protein, 8g carbohydrates, 20g fat, 6g saturated fat, 600mg sodium

87. BEEF AND PEA RISOTTO

Cooking time: 40 mins   **Yield:** 4

Ingredients

- 1 cup Arborio rice

- 1 pound lean ground beef
- 1 cup frozen peas
- 1 onion, diced
- 2 cloves garlic, minced
- 4 cups low-sodium beef broth
- 1/2 cup Parmesan cheese, grated
- 2 tablespoons olive oil
- 1/2 teaspoon salt
- 1/4 teaspoon black pepper

Instructions

- In a pot, sauté diced onion and minced garlic in olive oil until softened.
- Add lean ground beef and cook until browned.
- Stir in Arborio rice and cook for 2 minutes.
- Gradually add low-sodium beef broth, stirring frequently until the rice is creamy and cooked.
- Add frozen peas and grated Parmesan cheese, stirring until peas are heated through.
- Season with salt and black pepper.
- Serve the beef and pea risotto for a comforting and satisfying DASH Diet meal.

Nutritional Facts: 380 calories, 25g protein, 40g carbohydrates, 15g fat, 6g saturated fat, 600mg sodium

88. CHICKEN GINGER

Cooking time: 1 hr 35 mins   **Yield:** 4

Ingredients

- 1.5 pounds chicken thighs, bone-in and skin-on
- 2 tablespoons soy sauce (low-sodium)
- 1 tablespoon fresh ginger, grated
- 1 tablespoon honey
- 1 tablespoon rice vinegar
- 1 teaspoon sesame oil
- 1/2 teaspoon salt
- 1/4 teaspoon black pepper
- Chopped green onions for garnish

Instructions

- In a bowl, mix soy sauce, grated ginger, honey, rice vinegar, sesame oil, salt, and black pepper.
- Marinate chicken thighs in the mixture for at least 1 hour.
- Preheat the oven to 400°F (200°C).
- Roast chicken thighs for 20 minutes or until golden and cooked through.
- Garnish with chopped green onions and serve the flavorful chicken ginger for a zesty DASH Diet meal.

Nutritional Facts: 300 calories, 25g protein, 5g carbohydrates, 18g fat, 4.5g saturated fat, 600mg sodium

89.   TURKEY BBQ

Cooking time: 2hr 45mins   **Yield:** 4

Ingredients

- 1.5 pounds turkey breast, boneless and skinless
- 1 cup tomato sauce (low-sodium)
- 1/4 cup apple cider vinegar
- 2 tablespoons honey
- 1 tablespoon Worcestershire sauce
- 1 teaspoon smoked paprika
- 1/2 teaspoon salt
- 1/4 teaspoon black pepper

Instructions

- In a bowl, whisk together tomato sauce, apple cider vinegar, honey, Worcestershire sauce, smoked paprika, salt, and black pepper.
- Marinate turkey breast in the mixture for at least 2 hours.
- Preheat the grill to medium-high heat.
- Grill turkey breast for 25-30 minutes, turning occasionally, until fully cooked.
- Slice and serve the tangy turkey BBQ for a delicious DASH Diet meal.

Nutritional Facts: 280 calories, 30g protein, 10g carbohydrates, 8g fat, 1.5g saturated fat, 600mg sodium

90.   PORK WRAPS

Cooking time: 35mins   **Yield:** 4

Ingredients

- 1 pound pork tenderloin, sliced
- 1 cup shredded cabbage
- 1/2 cup shredded carrots
- 4 whole-grain tortillas
- 2 tablespoons hoisin sauce
- 1 tablespoon soy sauce (low-sodium)
- 1 tablespoon rice vinegar
- 1 teaspoon sesame oil
- 1/2 teaspoon salt
- 1/4 teaspoon black pepper

Instructions

- In a skillet, cook sliced pork tenderloin until browned and cooked through.
- In a bowl, mix hoisin sauce, soy sauce, rice vinegar, sesame oil, salt, and black pepper.
- Toss shredded cabbage and carrots in the sauce mixture.
- Warm whole-grain tortillas.
- Assemble pork slices and cabbage-carrot mix in the tortillas.
- Serve the pork wraps for a tasty and balanced DASH Diet meal.

Nutritional Facts: 320 calories, 25g protein, 30g carbohydrates, 12g fat, 3g saturated fat, 600mg sodium

CHAPTER 6

SEAFOOD & FISH OPTIONS

91.   PRAWNS PUTTANESCA

Cooking time: 35 mins   **Yield:** 4

Ingredients

- 1 pound large prawns, peeled and deveined
- 2 cups cherry tomatoes, halved
- 1/4 cup Kalamata olives, pitted and sliced
- 2 tablespoons capers
- 3 cloves garlic, minced
- 2 tablespoons olive oil
- 1 tablespoon tomato paste
- 1 teaspoon dried oregano
- 1/2 teaspoon red pepper flakes
- 1/2 teaspoon salt
- 1/4 teaspoon black pepper
- Fresh parsley for garnish

Instructions

- In a skillet, heat olive oil and sauté minced garlic until fragrant.
- Add cherry tomatoes, Kalamata olives, capers, tomato paste, dried oregano, red pepper flakes, salt, and black pepper.
- Cook the sauce for 10 minutes until tomatoes are softened.
- Add prawns and cook for an additional 5-7 minutes until prawns are pink and cooked through.
- Garnish with fresh parsley and serve the flavorful prawns puttanesca for a Mediterranean-inspired DASH Diet meal.

Nutritional Information (per serving): 280 calories, 25g protein, 12g carbohydrates, 15g fat, 2.5g saturated fat, 900mg sodium

92.   CRUNCHY BAKED FISH

Cooking time: 35 mins   **Yield:** 4

Ingredients

- 1.5 pounds white fish fillets (e.g., cod or tilapia)
- 1 cup whole wheat breadcrumbs
- 1/4 cup Parmesan cheese, grated
- 1 teaspoon dried thyme
- 1/2 teaspoon garlic powder
- 1/2 teaspoon paprika
- 1/2 teaspoon salt
- 1/4 teaspoon black pepper
- Olive oil spray

Instructions

- Adjust the oven temperature to 400°F (200°C) and place parchment paper on a baking pan.
- In a bowl, mix whole wheat breadcrumbs, Parmesan cheese, dried thyme, garlic powder, paprika, salt, and black pepper.
- Dip fish fillets in the breadcrumb mixture, coating evenly.
- Place coated fish on the prepared baking sheet.
- Lightly spray the top of the fish with olive oil spray.
- Bake for 20 minutes or until the fish is golden brown and cooked through.
- Serve the crunchy baked fish for a light and crispy DASH Diet meal.

Nutritional Information (per serving): 260 calories, 30g protein, 15g carbohydrates, 10g fat, 2.5g saturated fat, 600mg sodium

93.   ROASTED SALMON

Cooking time: 25 mins   **Yield:** 4

Ingredients

- 1.5 pounds salmon fillets
- 2 tablespoons Dijon mustard
- 1 tablespoon honey
- 1 tablespoon olive oil
- 1 teaspoon dried dill
- 1/2 teaspoon garlic powder
- 1/2 teaspoon salt

- 1/4 teaspoon black pepper
- Lemon wedges for serving

Instructions

- Adjust the oven temperature to 400°F (200°C) and place parchment paper on a baking pan.
- In a bowl, whisk together Dijon mustard, honey, olive oil, dried dill, garlic powder, salt, and black pepper.
- Put the salmon fillets onto the baking sheet that has been prepared.
- Brush the mustard-honey mixture over the top of the salmon.
- Bake for 15 minutes or until the salmon is flaky and cooked to your liking.
- Serve the roasted salmon with lemon wedges for a delightful and nutritious DASH Diet meal.

Nutritional Information (per serving): 320 calories, 30g protein, 10g carbohydrates, 18g fat, 3.5g saturated fat, 500mg sodium

94.   CRUNCHY TILAPIA WITH MANGO SALSA

Cooking time: 30mins   **Yield:** 4

Ingredients

- 1.5 pounds tilapia fillets
- 1 cup whole wheat breadcrumbs
- 1/4 cup unsweetened coconut flakes

- 1 teaspoon cumin
- 1/2 teaspoon garlic powder
- 1/2 teaspoon paprika
- 1/2 teaspoon salt
- 1/4 teaspoon black pepper
- Olive oil spray

Mango Salsa

- 1 ripe mango, diced
- 1/2 red onion, finely chopped
- 1/4 cup fresh cilantro, chopped
- Juice of 1 lime

Instructions

- Adjust the oven temperature to 400°F (200°C) and place parchment paper on a baking pan.
- In a bowl, mix whole wheat breadcrumbs, coconut flakes, cumin, garlic powder, paprika, salt, and black pepper.
- Coat tilapia fillets with the breadcrumb mixture and place them on the prepared baking sheet.
- Lightly spray the top of the tilapia with olive oil spray.
- Bake for 15 minutes or until the tilapia is crispy and cooked through.
- In a separate bowl, combine diced mango, chopped red onion, fresh cilantro, and lime juice to make the salsa.
- Serve the crunchy tilapia topped with mango salsa for a tropical and nutritious DASH Diet meal.

Nutritional Information (per serving): 290 calories, 30g protein, 20g carbohydrates, 12g fat, 4g saturated fat, 600mg sodium

95. SEAFOOD CORN CHOWDER

Cooking time: 45 mins   **Yield:** 6

Ingredients

- 1 pound mixed seafood (shrimp, scallops, and/or white fish)
- 2 cups corn kernels (fresh or frozen)
- 1 onion, finely chopped
- 2 potatoes, diced
- 2 carrots, diced
- 3 cups low-sodium vegetable broth
- 1 cup 2% milk
- 2 tablespoons olive oil
- 1 teaspoon thyme
- 1/2 teaspoon smoked paprika
- 1/2 teaspoon salt
- 1/4 teaspoon black pepper
- Chopped fresh parsley for garnish

Instructions

- In a pot, sauté chopped onion in olive oil until softened.

- Add diced potatoes, carrots, thyme, smoked paprika, salt, and black pepper.
- Pour in vegetable broth and bring to a simmer until potatoes are tender.
- Add mixed seafood and corn kernels, cooking until seafood is cooked through.
- Pour in milk, stir, and simmer for an additional 5 minutes.
- Garnish with chopped fresh parsley and serve the hearty seafood corn chowder for a comforting DASH Diet meal.

Nutritional Information (per serving): 280 calories, 25g protein, 35g carbohydrates, 8g fat, 2g saturated fat, 600mg sodium

96. BAKED LEMON SALMON

Cooking time: 25mins   **Yield:** 4

Ingredients

- 1.5 pounds salmon fillets
- Zest and juice of 1 lemon
- 2 tablespoons olive oil
- 1 teaspoon dried dill
- 1/2 teaspoon garlic powder
- 1/2 teaspoon salt
- 1/4 teaspoon black pepper
- Lemon slices for garnish

Instructions

- Adjust the oven temperature to 400°F (200°C) and place parchment paper on a baking pan.
- In a bowl, whisk together lemon zest, lemon juice, olive oil, dried dill, garlic powder, salt, and black pepper.
- Put the salmon fillets onto the baking sheet that has been prepared.
- Pour the lemon mixture over the top of the salmon.
- Bake for 15 minutes or until the salmon is flaky and cooked to your liking.
- Garnish with lemon slices and serve the baked lemon salmon for a fresh and flavorful DASH Diet meal.

Nutritional Information (per serving): 320 calories, 30g protein, 3g carbohydrates, 20g fat, 3.5g saturated fat, 500mg sodium

97. CAJUN SHRIMP

Cooking time: 15 mins   **Yield:** 4

Ingredients

- 1 pound large shrimp, peeled and deveined
- 2 tablespoons Cajun seasoning
- 1 tablespoon olive oil
- 1/2 teaspoon salt
- 1/4 teaspoon black pepper
- Fresh parsley for garnish
- Lemon wedges for serving

Instructions

- In a bowl, toss shrimp with Cajun seasoning, olive oil, salt, and black pepper.
- Heat a skillet over medium-high heat.
- Cook shrimp for 2-3 minutes per side or until pink and opaque.
- Garnish with fresh parsley and serve with lemon wedges for a zesty DASH Diet meal.

Nutritional Information (per serving): 180 calories, 25g protein, 2g carbohydrates, 8g fat, 1.5g saturated fat, 600mg sodium

98.   BAKED COD WITH LEMON PEPPER SAUCE

Cooking time: 35 mins   **Yield:** 4

Ingredients

- 1.5 pounds cod fillets
- 2 tablespoons olive oil
- Zest and juice of 1 lemon
- 1 teaspoon dried thyme
- 1/2 teaspoon garlic powder
- 1/2 teaspoon black pepper
- 1/2 teaspoon salt
- Fresh dill for garnish
- Lemon Pepper Sauce
- 1/4 cup Greek yogurt (low-fat)
- 1 teaspoon lemon zest
- 1 tablespoon lemon juice

- 1/2 teaspoon black pepper
- 1/4 teaspoon salt

Instructions

- Adjust the oven temperature to 400°F (200°C) and place parchment paper on a baking pan.
- In a bowl, mix olive oil, lemon zest, lemon juice, dried thyme, garlic powder, black pepper, and salt.
- Coat cod fillets with the mixture and place them on the prepared baking sheet.
- Bake for 20 minutes or until the cod is flaky and cooked through.
- In a small bowl, whisk together Greek yogurt, lemon zest, lemon juice, black pepper, and salt to make the sauce.
- Garnish the baked cod with fresh dill and serve with lemon pepper sauce for a light and flavorful DASH Diet meal.

Nutritional Information (per serving): 250 calories, 30g protein, 3g carbohydrates, 12g fat, 2g saturated fat, 600mg sodium

99.   OVEN BAKED TILAPIA

Cooking time: 25 mins   **Yield:** 6

Ingredients

- 1.5 pounds tilapia fillets
- 2 tablespoons olive oil
- 1 teaspoon dried basil

- 1/2 teaspoon garlic powder
- 1/2 teaspoon onion powder
- 1/2 teaspoon black pepper
- 1/2 teaspoon salt
- Lemon wedges for serving

Instructions

- Adjust the oven temperature to 400°F (200°C) and place parchment paper on a baking pan.
- In a bowl, mix olive oil, dried basil, garlic powder, onion powder, black pepper, and salt.
- Coat tilapia fillets with the mixture and place them on the prepared baking sheet.
- Bake for 15 minutes or until the tilapia is flaky and cooked through.
- Serve with lemon wedges for a simple and satisfying DASH Diet meal.

Nutritional Information (per serving): 220 calories, 25g protein, 0g carbohydrates, 12g fat, 2g saturated fat, 500mg sodium

100. FISH TACOS

Cooking time: 30 mins   **Yield:** 4

Ingredients

- 1 pound white fish fillets (cod or tilapia)
- 2 tablespoons olive oil
- 1 tablespoon taco seasoning

- 1/2 teaspoon cumin
- 1/2 teaspoon paprika
- 1/2 teaspoon garlic powder
- 1/2 teaspoon salt
- 1/4 teaspoon black pepper
- Whole-grain tortillas
- Cabbage slaw (shredded cabbage, carrots, Greek yogurt, lime juice)
- Avocado slices for garnish
- Fresh cilantro for garnish

Instructions

- In a bowl, mix olive oil, taco seasoning, cumin, paprika, garlic powder, salt, and black pepper.
- Coat fish fillets with the mixture and cook in a skillet over medium-high heat until fully cooked.
- Warm whole-grain tortillas.
- Assemble tacos with cooked fish, cabbage slaw, avocado slices, and fresh cilantro.
- Serve the fish tacos for a flavorful and balanced DASH Diet meal.

Nutritional Information (per serving): 320 calories, 25g protein, 30g carbohydrates, 15g fat, 2.5g saturated fat, 600mg sodium

101. TUNA BROCCOLI PASTA

Cooking time: 30 mins   **Yield:** 4

Ingredients

- 8 ounces whole-grain pasta
- Two drained cans (5 ounces each) of tuna in water
- 2 cups broccoli florets
- 2 tablespoons olive oil
- 2 cloves garlic, minced
- 1/2 teaspoon red pepper flakes
- 1/2 teaspoon dried basil
- 1/2 teaspoon salt
- 1/4 teaspoon black pepper
- Grated Parmesan cheese for garnish

Instructions

- Cook whole-grain pasta according to package instructions, adding broccoli in the last 3 minutes of cooking.
- In a skillet, sauté minced garlic in olive oil until fragrant.
- Add drained tuna, red pepper flakes, dried basil, salt, and black pepper. Cook for 3-5 minutes.
- Combine the tuna mixture with cooked pasta and broccoli.
- Garnish with grated Parmesan cheese and serve the tuna broccoli pasta for a protein-packed DASH Diet meal.

Nutritional Information (per serving): 380 calories, 30g protein, 45g carbohydrates, 12g fat, 2g saturated fat, 600mg sodium

102. SPICY SHRIMP STIR FRY WITH BROWN RICE

Cooking time: 25 mins   **Yield:** 4

Ingredients

- 1 pound large shrimp, peeled and deveined
- 2 cups broccoli florets
- 1 bell pepper, sliced
- 1 cup snap peas
- 2 tablespoons soy sauce (low-sodium)
- 1 tablespoon hoisin sauce
- 1 tablespoon olive oil
- 1 teaspoon Sriracha sauce (adjust to taste)
- 1/2 teaspoon ginger, grated
- 1/2 teaspoon garlic, minced
- 1/2 teaspoon salt
- 1/4 teaspoon black pepper
- Cooked brown rice for serving

Instructions

- In a bowl, mix soy sauce, hoisin sauce, Sriracha sauce, grated ginger, minced garlic, salt, and black pepper.
- In a wok or skillet, heat olive oil and stir-fry shrimp until pink and opaque.
- Add broccoli, bell pepper, and snap peas. Stir-fry until vegetables are tender-crisp.
- Pour the sauce over the shrimp and vegetables, tossing to coat evenly.

- Serve the spicy shrimp stir fry over cooked brown rice for a vibrant and savory DASH Diet meal.

Nutritional Information (per serving): 290 calories, 25g protein, 30g carbohydrates, 8g fat, 1.5g saturated fat, 600mg sodium

103.   GRILLED VEGETABLE AND HALLOUMI SKEWERS

Cooking time: 30mins   **Yield:** 4

Ingredients

- 1 zucchini, sliced
- 1 bell pepper, cut into chunks
- 1 red onion, cut into wedges
- 8 cherry tomatoes
- 8 ounces halloumi cheese, cut into cubes
- 2 tablespoons olive oil
- 1 teaspoon dried oregano
- 1/2 teaspoon garlic powder
- 1/2 teaspoon black pepper
- 1/2 teaspoon salt
- Wooden skewers, soaked in water

Instructions

- Preheat the grill to medium-high heat.
- In a bowl, toss zucchini, bell pepper, red onion, cherry tomatoes, and halloumi cubes with olive oil, dried oregano, garlic powder, black pepper, and salt.

- Thread the vegetables and halloumi onto soaked wooden skewers.
- Grill skewers for 5 minutes per side or until vegetables are tender and halloumi is lightly browned.
- Serve the grilled vegetable and halloumi skewers for a flavorful and nutritious DASH Diet meal.

Nutritional Information (per serving): 280 calories, 15g protein, 15g carbohydrates, 18g fat, 8g saturated fat, 700mg sodium

104.   TUNA SALAD LETTUCE WRAPS

Cooking time: 15 mins   **Yield:** 4

Ingredients

- Two drained cans (5 ounces each) of tuna in water
- 1/2 cup Greek yogurt (low-fat)
- 1 celery stalk, finely chopped
- 1/4 red onion, finely chopped
- 1 tablespoon Dijon mustard
- 1 tablespoon lemon juice
- 1/2 teaspoon dried dill
- 1/2 teaspoon black pepper
- 1/4 teaspoon salt
- Butter lettuce leaves for wrapping

Instructions

- In a bowl, mix tuna, Greek yogurt, chopped celery, red onion, Dijon mustard, lemon juice, dried dill, black pepper, and salt.

- Spoon the tuna salad onto butter lettuce leaves, creating wraps.
- Serve the tuna salad lettuce wraps for a light and protein-rich DASH Diet meal.

Nutritional Information (per serving): 220 calories, 25g protein, 5g carbohydrates, 10g fat, 2g saturated fat, 600mg sodium

105. SHRIMP AND QUINOA STIR FRY

Cooking time: 30mins   **Yield:** 4

Ingredients

- 1 pound large shrimp, peeled and deveined
- 1 cup quinoa, cooked
- 2 cups broccoli florets
- 1 bell pepper, sliced
- 1 carrot, julienned
- 2 tablespoons soy sauce (low-sodium)
- 1 tablespoon hoisin sauce
- 1 tablespoon olive oil
- 1 teaspoon ginger, grated
- 1/2 teaspoon garlic, minced
- 1/2 teaspoon Sriracha sauce (adjust to taste)
- 1/2 teaspoon salt
- 1/4 teaspoon black pepper

Instructions

- In a bowl, mix soy sauce, hoisin sauce, grated ginger, minced garlic, Sriracha sauce, salt, and black pepper.
- In a wok or skillet, heat olive oil and stir-fry shrimp until pink and opaque.
- Add broccoli, bell pepper, and julienned carrot. Stir-fry until vegetables are tender-crisp.
- Add cooked quinoa and the sauce, tossing to coat evenly.
- Serve the shrimp and quinoa stir fry for a wholesome and flavorful DASH Diet meal.

Nutritional Information (per serving): 320 calories, 25g protein, 35g carbohydrates, 10g fat, 1.5g saturated fat, 600mg sodium

CHAPTER 7

SNACKS AND SIDE DISHES

106. CUCUMBER AND TOMATO SALAD

Cooking time: 10 mins   **Yield:** 4

Ingredients

- 2 cucumbers, sliced
- 2 cups cherry tomatoes, halved
- 1/2 red onion, thinly sliced
- 1/4 cup feta cheese, crumbled
- 2 tablespoons olive oil
- 1 tablespoon red wine vinegar
- 1 teaspoon dried oregano
- 1/2 teaspoon black pepper
- 1/2 teaspoon salt
- Fresh basil for garnish

Instructions

- In a bowl, combine sliced cucumbers, halved cherry tomatoes, thinly sliced red onion, and crumbled feta cheese.
- In a small bowl, whisk together olive oil, red wine vinegar, dried oregano, black pepper, and salt.
- Drizzle the salad with the dressing and toss to coat.
- Garnish with fresh basil and serve the cucumber and tomato salad for a refreshing and low-sodium DASH Diet side dish.

Nutritional Information (per serving): 120 calories, 3g protein, 10g carbohydrates, 8g fat, 2.5g saturated fat, 400mg sodium

107. GREEK SALAD SKEWERS

Cooking time: 20 mins   **Yield:** 4

Ingredients

- 1 cup cherry tomatoes
- 1 cucumber, cut into chunks
- 1 cup Kalamata olives, pitted
- 1 cup feta cheese, cubed
- 1 tablespoon olive oil
- 1 tablespoon red wine vinegar
- 1 teaspoon dried oregano
- 1/2 teaspoon black pepper
- 1/2 teaspoon salt
- Wooden skewers

Instructions

- Thread cherry tomatoes, cucumber chunks, Kalamata olives, and feta cheese onto wooden skewers.
- In a small bowl, whisk together olive oil, red wine vinegar, dried oregano, black pepper, and salt.
- Drizzle the dressing over the skewers.

- Serve the Greek salad skewers for a delightful and low-sodium DASH Diet appetizer or side.

Nutritional Information (per serving): 180 calories, 5g protein, 8g carbohydrates, 15g fat, 7g saturated fat, 500mg sodium

108.   KALE CHIPS

Cooking time: 25 mins   **Yield:** 4

Ingredients

- One bunch of chopped and shredded kale (without stems)
- 1 tablespoon olive oil
- 1/2 teaspoon garlic powder
- 1/2 teaspoon onion powder
- 1/2 teaspoon paprika
- 1/2 teaspoon black pepper
- 1/4 teaspoon salt

Instructions

- Adjust the oven temperature to 350°F (175°C) and place parchment paper on a baking pan.
- In a bowl, toss kale pieces with olive oil, garlic powder, onion powder, paprika, black pepper, and salt.
- Spread the kale on the prepared baking sheet in a single layer.
- Bake the kale for 15 minutes, or until it becomes crispy.

- Allow to cool before serving the kale chips as a crunchy and nutritious DASH Diet snack.

Nutritional Information (per serving): 70 calories, 3g protein, 7g carbohydrates, 4.5g fat, 0.5g saturated fat, 200mg sodium

109.   SLICED APPLE WITH ALMOND BUTTER

Cooking time: 5 mins   **Yield:** 4

Ingredients

- 2 apples, thinly sliced
- 4 tablespoons almond butter
- 1 teaspoon honey (optional)
- 1/4 teaspoon cinnamon

Instructions

- On a serving platter, arrange the apple slices.
- In a small bowl, mix almond butter with honey (if using), cinnamon, and a pinch of salt.
- Serve the almond butter mixture alongside the sliced apples for a wholesome and satisfying DASH Diet snack.

Nutritional Information (per serving): 220 calories, 4g protein, 30g carbohydrates, 11g fat, 1g saturated fat, 80mg sodium

110. CAULIFLOWER POPCORN

Cooking time: 30mins   **Yield**: 4

Ingredients

- 1 head cauliflower, cut into florets
- 2 tablespoons olive oil
- 1 teaspoon garlic powder
- 1/2 teaspoon onion powder
- 1/2 teaspoon paprika
- 1/2 teaspoon black pepper
- 1/4 teaspoon salt

Instructions

- Adjust the oven temperature to 400°F (200°C) and place parchment paper on a baking pan.
- In a bowl, toss cauliflower florets with olive oil, garlic powder, onion powder, paprika, black pepper, and salt.
- Spread the cauliflower on the prepared baking sheet in a single layer.
- Bake for 20 minutes or until the cauliflower is golden brown and crispy.
- Serve the cauliflower popcorn for a flavorful and low-sodium DASH Diet snack.

Nutritional Information (per serving): 80 calories, 3g protein, 10g carbohydrates, 4.5g fat, 0.5g saturated fat, 180mg sodium

111. AVOCADO AND SALSA DIP

Cooking time: 10 mins   **Yield**: 4

Ingredients

- 2 avocados, peeled and mashed
- 1/2 cup salsa (no added salt)
- 1 tablespoon lime juice
- 1/2 teaspoon garlic powder
- 1/2 teaspoon onion powder
- 1/2 teaspoon cumin
- Pinch of salt

Instructions

- In a bowl, combine mashed avocados, salsa, lime juice, garlic powder, onion powder, cumin, and a pinch of salt.
- Stir thoroughly to ensure that all ingredients are equally mixed.
- Serve the avocado and salsa dip with whole-grain chips or fresh vegetables for a creamy and flavorful DASH Diet snack.

Nutritional Information (per serving): 150 calories, 2g protein, 12g carbohydrates, 11g fat, 1.5g saturated fat, 120mg sodium

112. SPINACH AND TOMATO FRITTATA

Cooking time: 30 mins   **Yield:** 4

Ingredients

- 6 large eggs
- 1 cup spinach, chopped
- 1 cup cherry tomatoes, halved
- 1/2 cup feta cheese, crumbled
- 1/4 cup red onion, finely chopped
- 1 tablespoon olive oil
- 1 teaspoon dried oregano
- 1/2 teaspoon garlic powder
- 1/2 teaspoon black pepper
- 1/4 teaspoon salt

Instructions

- Preheat the oven to 375°F (190°C).
- In a bowl, whisk together eggs, chopped spinach, cherry tomatoes, feta cheese, red onion, dried oregano, garlic powder, black pepper, and salt.
- Heat the olive oil in an ovenproof skillet over medium heat.
- Pour the egg mixture into the skillet and cook for 3-4 minutes until the edges begin to set.
- Transfer the skillet to the preheated oven and bake for 15-18 minutes until the frittata is set and slightly golden.
- Allow it to cool slightly, slice, and serve the spinach and tomato frittata for a protein-packed DASH Diet breakfast or brunch.

Nutritional Information (per serving): 220 calories, 14g protein, 7g carbohydrates, 16g fat, 6g saturated fat, 400mg sodium

113. CRISPY SHRIMP

Cooking time: 25 mins   **Yield:** 4

Ingredients

- 1 pound large shrimp, peeled and deveined
- 1 cup whole-wheat breadcrumbs
- 1 teaspoon paprika
- 1/2 teaspoon garlic powder
- 1/2 teaspoon onion powder
- 1/2 teaspoon black pepper
- 1/4 teaspoon salt
- 2 eggs, beaten
- Olive oil spray

Instructions

- Adjust the oven temperature to 425°F (220°C) and place parchment paper on a baking pan.
- In a bowl, mix whole-wheat breadcrumbs, paprika, garlic powder, onion powder, black pepper, and salt.
- Dip each shrimp in beaten eggs, then coat with the breadcrumb mixture.
- Put the coated shrimp onto the baking sheet that has been prepared.
- Spray the shrimp with olive oil spray.
- Bake for 8-10 minutes until the shrimp are golden and crispy.
- Serve the crispy shrimp for a tasty and low-sodium DASH Diet seafood dish.

Nutritional Information (per serving): 240 calories, 25g protein, 20g carbohydrates, 8g fat, 1.5g saturated fat, 350mg sodium

114. APPLE SNACK

Cooking time: 5 mins   **Yield:** 1

Ingredients

- 1 apple, sliced
- 2 tablespoons almond butter
- Cinnamon for sprinkling
- Pinch of salt

Instructions

- Arrange the sliced apples on a plate.
- Spread almond butter on the apple slices.
- Sprinkle with cinnamon and add a pinch of salt.
- Serve the apple snack for a quick and satisfying DASH Diet treat.

Nutritional Information (per serving): 220 calories, 3g protein, 30g carbohydrates, 11g fat, 1g saturated fat, 50mg sodium

115. POTATO CRISP

Cooking time: 15 mins   **Yield:** 4

Ingredients

- 4 large potatoes, thinly sliced
- 2 tablespoons olive oil

- 1 teaspoon paprika
- 1/2 teaspoon garlic powder
- 1/2 teaspoon onion powder
- 1/2 teaspoon black pepper
- 1/4 teaspoon salt

Instructions

- Before proceeding, preheat the oven to 375°F (190°C) and place parchment paper on a baking pan.
- In a bowl, toss thinly sliced potatoes with olive oil, paprika, garlic powder, onion powder, black pepper, and salt.
- Arrange the seasoned potato slices on the prepared baking sheet in a single layer.
- Bake for 20-25 minutes or until the potatoes are golden and crispy.
- Allow to cool slightly before serving the potato crisps as a savory and low-sodium DASH Diet snack.

Nutritional Information (per serving): 180 calories, 3g protein, 30g carbohydrates, 6g fat, 1g saturated fat, 150mg sodium

116. LENTIL MEDLEY

Cooking time: 35 mins   **Yield:** 4

Ingredients

- 1 cup dried green lentils
- 2 cups vegetable broth (low-sodium)
- 1 cup cherry tomatoes, halved

- 1/2 cup cucumber, diced
- 1/4 cup red onion, finely chopped
- 2 tablespoons fresh parsley, chopped
- 2 tablespoons olive oil
- 1 tablespoon balsamic vinegar
- 1 teaspoon Dijon mustard
- 1/2 teaspoon black pepper
- 1/4 teaspoon salt

Instructions

- Rinse lentils under cold water and place them in a saucepan with vegetable broth. Bring to a boil, then simmer for 20-25 minutes or until lentils are tender.
- In a large bowl, combine cooked lentils, cherry tomatoes, diced cucumber, red onion, and fresh parsley.
- In a small bowl, whisk together olive oil, balsamic vinegar, Dijon mustard, black pepper, and salt.
- Pour the dressing over the lentil medley and toss to combine.
- Serve the lentil medley as a protein-packed and flavorful DASH Diet side dish.

Nutritional Information (per serving): 220 calories, 12g protein, 32g carbohydrates, 6g fat, 1g saturated fat, 200mg sodium

117. SPICY ALMONDS

Cooking time: 20 mins   **Yield:** 4

Ingredients

- 2 cups raw almonds
- 1 tablespoon olive oil
- 1 teaspoon chili powder
- 1/2 teaspoon cayenne pepper
- 1/2 teaspoon garlic powder
- 1/2 teaspoon onion powder
- 1/4 teaspoon salt

Instructions

- Adjust the oven temperature to 350°F (175°C) and place parchment paper on a baking pan.
- In a bowl, toss raw almonds with olive oil, chili powder, cayenne pepper, garlic powder, onion powder, and salt.
- Spread the seasoned almonds on the prepared baking sheet in a single layer.
- Roast for 12-15 minutes or until the almonds are fragrant and lightly toasted.
- Allow to cool before serving the spicy almonds as a crunchy and satisfying DASH Diet snack.

Nutritional Information (per serving): 240 calories, 9g protein, 9g carbohydrates, 20g fat, 2g saturated fat, 150mg sodium

118. CILANTRO LIME SHRIMP

Cooking time: 22 mins   **Yield:** 2

Ingredients

- 1 pound large shrimp, peeled and deveined
- 2 tablespoons olive oil
- 3 cloves garlic, minced
- Zest and juice of 2 limes
- 1/4 cup fresh cilantro, chopped
- 1 teaspoon cumin
- 1/2 teaspoon chili powder
- 1/2 teaspoon black pepper
- 1/4 teaspoon salt

Instructions

- In a bowl, combine shrimp with olive oil, minced garlic, lime zest, lime juice, chopped cilantro, cumin, chili powder, black pepper, and salt.
- Heat a skillet over medium-high heat.
- Add the shrimp mixture to the skillet and cook for 2-3 minutes per side until the shrimp are opaque and cooked through.
- Serve the cilantro lime shrimp as a zesty and low-sodium DASH Diet seafood dish.

Nutritional Information (per serving): 200 calories, 20g protein, 2g carbohydrates, 12g fat, 1.5g saturated fat, 250mg sodium

119. QUINOA ENERGY BALLS

Cooking time: 45 mins   **Yield:** 12

Ingredients

- 1 cup cooked quinoa, cooled
- 1/2 cup almond butter
- 1/4 cup honey
- 1/2 cup rolled oats
- 1/4 cup chia seeds
- 1/4 cup dark chocolate chips
- 1 teaspoon vanilla extract
- 1/4 teaspoon salt

Instructions

- In a bowl, combine cooked quinoa, almond butter, honey, rolled oats, chia seeds, dark chocolate chips, vanilla extract, and salt.
- Mix until well combined.
- Refrigerate the mixture for 30 minutes.
- Shape into bite-sized energy balls.
- Serve the quinoa energy balls as a wholesome and low-sodium DASH Diet snack.

Nutritional Information (per serving): 120 calories, 4g protein, 14g carbohydrates, 6g fat, 1g saturated fat, 50mg sodium

120. ASPARAGUS AND TOMATO QUICHE

Cooking time: 10 mins   **Yield:** 4

Ingredients

- 2 cups mixed vegetable sticks (carrots, cucumber, bell peppers)

- 1 cup hummus (low-sodium)
- 1 tablespoon olive oil
- 1/2 teaspoon paprika
- 1/4 teaspoon salt

Instructions

- Arrange mixed vegetable sticks on a serving plate.
- In a small bowl, mix hummus with olive oil, paprika, and salt.
- Serve the veggie sticks with hummus for a crunchy and flavorful DASH Diet snack.

Nutritional Information (per serving): 150 calories, 6g protein, 15g carbohydrates, 8g fat, 1g saturated fat, 200mg sodium

Chapter 8

Desserts with a DASH Twist

121. Yogurt with Fresh Strawberries and Honey

Cooking time: 5 mins   **Yield:** 2

Ingredients

- 1 cup low-fat Greek yogurt
- 1 cup fresh strawberries, sliced
- 2 tablespoons honey
- 1/2 teaspoon vanilla extract
- Pinch of salt

Instructions

- In serving bowls, divide the Greek yogurt.
- Top each bowl with sliced fresh strawberries.
- Drizzle with honey and add a splash of vanilla extract.
- Sprinkle a pinch of salt for balance.
- Serve the yogurt with fresh strawberries and honey for a delightful and low-sodium DASH Diet breakfast or snack.

Nutritional Information (per serving): 150 calories, 10g protein, 25g carbohydrates, 2g fat, 1g saturated fat, 50mg sodium

122. Light Pumpkin Pie

Cooking time: 2 hr 55 mins   **Yield:** 8

Ingredients

- 1 can (15 ounces) pumpkin puree
- 1/2 cup unsweetened applesauce
- 1/2 cup non-fat Greek yogurt
- 2 eggs
- 1/2 cup honey
- 1 teaspoon cinnamon
- 1/2 teaspoon nutmeg
- 1/2 teaspoon ginger
- 1/4 teaspoon salt
- 1 pre-made whole-wheat pie crust

Instructions

- Preheat the oven to 350°F (175°C).
- In a bowl, mix pumpkin puree, applesauce, Greek yogurt, eggs, honey, cinnamon, nutmeg, ginger, and salt until well combined.
- Fill the whole-wheat pie crust with the ingredients.
- Bake the pie for 40 minutes, or until it sets.
- Before serving, let the pie cool and then place it in the refrigerator for at least two hours.

- Slice and enjoy the light pumpkin pie as a flavorful and low-sodium DASH Diet dessert.

Nutritional Information (per serving): 220 calories, 5g protein, 40g carbohydrates, 6g fat, 2g saturated fat, 180mg sodium

123. TAHINI AND ALMOND COOKIES

Cooking time: 27 mins   **Yield:** 12

Ingredients

- 1 cup almond flour
- 1/4 cup tahini
- 1/4 cup honey
- 1 egg
- 1/2 teaspoon vanilla extract
- 1/4 teaspoon baking soda
- Pinch of salt

Instructions

- Adjust the oven temperature to 350°F (175°C) and place parchment paper on a baking pan.
- In a bowl, mix almond flour, tahini, honey, egg, vanilla extract, baking soda, and a pinch of salt until a dough forms.
- Scoop out dough in tablespoon-sized parts, then roll them into balls. Transfer them on the baking sheet that's been ready.

- Using a fork, gently flatten each ball to make a crosshatch design.
- Bake for 12 minutes, or until brown around the edges.
- Allow the cookies to cool before serving the tahini and almond cookies as a nutty and low-sodium DASH Diet treat.

Nutritional Information (per serving): 120 calories, 3g protein, 10g carbohydrates, 8g fat, 0.5g saturated fat, 50mg sodium

124. OATMEAL WALNUT CHOCOLATE CHIP COOKIES

Cooking time: 27 mins   **Yield:** 2

Ingredients

- 1 cup old-fashioned oats
- 3/4 cup whole wheat flour
- 1/2 cup chopped walnuts
- 1/2 cup dark chocolate chips
- 1/2 cup unsalted butter, softened
- 1/2 cup honey
- 1 large egg
- 1 teaspoon vanilla extract
- 1/2 teaspoon baking soda
- 1/4 teaspoon salt

Instructions

- Adjust the oven temperature to 350°F (175°C) and place parchment paper on a baking pan.

- In a bowl, combine oats, whole wheat flour, chopped walnuts, and dark chocolate chips.
- In another bowl, cream together softened butter and honey until smooth. Mix thoroughly after adding the egg and vanilla essence.
- Stirring until well blended, gradually add the dry ingredients to the wet ones.
- Drop dough onto the baking sheet that has been prepared in tablespoon-sized pieces.
- Bake until the edges turn brown, 10 to 12 minutes.
- Allow the cookies to cool on a wire rack before serving the oatmeal walnut chocolate chip cookies as a delightful and low-sodium DASH Diet dessert.

Nutritional Information (per serving): 110 calories, 2g protein, 13g carbohydrates, 6g fat, 2.5g saturated fat, 50mg sodium

125. PEAR-CRANBERRY PIE WITH OATMEAL STREUSEL

Cooking time: 1 hr 10 mins   **Yield:** 8

Ingredients

- 5 cups sliced ripe pears
- 1 cup fresh cranberries
- 1/4 cup honey
- 2 tablespoons whole wheat flour
- 1 teaspoon cinnamon
- 1/2 teaspoon nutmeg
- 1/4 teaspoon salt
- Oatmeal streusel topping (1/2 cup oats, 1/4 cup whole wheat flour, 2 tablespoons honey, 2 tablespoons unsalted butter, 1/4 teaspoon salt)

Instructions

- Preheat the oven to 375°F (190°C) and place a pie crust in a pie dish.
- In a large bowl, mix sliced pears, fresh cranberries, honey, whole wheat flour, cinnamon, nutmeg, and salt.
- Spoon the fruit mixture into the pie crust.
- In a separate bowl, combine oats, whole wheat flour, honey, softened unsalted butter, and salt to create the oatmeal streusel.
- Sprinkle the streusel over the fruit mixture.
- Bake for 50 minutes or until the filling is bubbly, and the streusel is golden.
- Allow the pie to cool before serving the pear-cranberry pie with oatmeal streusel as a fruity and low-sodium DASH Diet dessert.

Nutritional Information (per serving): 250 calories, 2g protein, 40g carbohydrates, 10g fat, 4g saturated fat, 120mg sodium

126. MILK CHOCOLATE PUDDING

Cooking time: 2 hr 20 min   **Yield:** 4

Ingredients

- 3 tablespoons cornstarch
- 1/4 cup unsweetened cocoa powder
- 1/2 cup honey
- 2 1/2 cups low-fat milk
- 1/2 cup milk chocolate chips
- 1 teaspoon vanilla extract
- 1/4 teaspoon salt

Instructions

- In a bowl, whisk together cornstarch, cocoa powder, and honey.
- In a saucepan, heat low-fat milk over medium heat until warm.
- Gradually whisk the dry ingredients into the warm milk, stirring constantly until the mixture thickens.
- Add milk chocolate chips, vanilla extract, and salt. Continue stirring until the chocolate chips are melted.
- Take it off the fire and let it to cool a little.
- Pour the pudding into serving bowls and refrigerate for at least 2 hours before serving the milk chocolate pudding as a creamy and low-sodium DASH Diet dessert.

Nutritional Information (per serving): 220 calories, 6g protein, 40g carbohydrates, 5g fat, 3g saturated fat, 80mg sodium

127. LIGHT AND EASY PEAR-STRAWBERRY TRIFLE

Cooking time: 1hrs 15mins   **Yield:** 6

Ingredients

- 2 ripe pears, diced
- 1 cup fresh strawberries, sliced
- 1 cup low-fat vanilla yogurt
- 1/2 cup angel food cake, cubed
- 1/4 cup honey
- 1 teaspoon vanilla extract
- 1/4 teaspoon salt

Instructions

- In a bowl, mix diced pears and sliced strawberries.
- In another bowl, combine low-fat vanilla yogurt, cubed angel food cake, honey, vanilla extract, and salt.
- In serving glasses, layer the fruit mixture and yogurt mixture.
- Layers should be repeated until the glasses are full.
- Refrigerate for at least 1 hour before serving the light and easy pear-strawberry trifle as a refreshing and low-sodium DASH Diet dessert.

Nutritional Information (per serving): 120 calories, 2g protein, 25g carbohydrates, 1g fat, 0.5g saturated fat, 75mg sodium

128. GUILT-FREE BANANA BERRY ICE CREAM

Cooking time: 4 hrs 5 mins   **Yields:** 4

Ingredients

- 3 ripe bananas, sliced and frozen
- 1 cup mixed berries (strawberries, blueberries, raspberries)
- 1/2 cup low-fat milk
- 1 tablespoon honey
- 1 teaspoon vanilla extract
- 1/4 teaspoon salt

Instructions

- In a blender, combine frozen banana slices, mixed berries, low-fat milk, honey, vanilla extract, and salt.
- Blend until smooth and creamy.
- After transferring the mixture into a loaf pan, freeze it for a minimum of four hours.
- Scoop and serve the guilt-free banana berry ice cream as a satisfying and low-sodium DASH Diet frozen treat.

Nutritional Information (per serving): 100 calories, 1g protein, 25g carbohydrates, 0.5g fat, 0g saturated fat, 50mg sodium

129. FABULOUS FIG BARS

Cooking time: 1 hr 45 mins   **Yield:** 12

Ingredients

- 1 cup dried figs, stems removed
- 1/2 cup boiling water
- 1 cup old-fashioned oats
- 1/2 cup whole wheat flour
- 1/4 cup honey
- 2 tablespoons unsalted butter, melted
- 1 teaspoon vanilla extract
- 1/4 teaspoon salt

Instructions

- Adjust the oven temperature to 350°F (175°C) and place parchment paper in a baking dish.
- In a bowl, soak dried figs in boiling water for 10 minutes, then drain.
- In a food processor, blend figs until smooth.
- In a separate bowl, mix old-fashioned oats, whole wheat flour, honey, melted unsalted butter, vanilla extract, and salt.
- Half of the oat mixture should be pressed into the baking dish's bottom.
- Cover the crust with the fig purée.
- Scatter the leftover oat mixture on top of the layer of figs.
- Bake until the top is brown, about 25 minutes.

- Allow the bars to cool before cutting and serving the fabulous fig bars as a wholesome and low-sodium DASH Diet snack.

Nutritional Information (per serving): 130 calories, 2g protein, 25g carbohydrates, 3g fat, 1.5g saturated fat, 50mg sodium

130. CALIFORNIA SKINNY DIPS

Cooking time: 30 mins   **Yield:** 8

Ingredients

- 1 cup low-fat Greek yogurt
- 1 ripe avocado, mashed
- 1/2 cup diced cucumber
- 1/4 cup chopped fresh cilantro
- 1 tablespoon lime juice
- 1/2 teaspoon garlic powder
- 1/4 teaspoon salt

Instructions

- In a bowl, combine low-fat Greek yogurt and mashed avocado until smooth.
- Stir in diced cucumber, chopped cilantro, lime juice, garlic powder, and salt.
- After thoroughly mixing, let it chill for at least one hour.
- Serve the California Skinny Dips with fresh vegetables or whole-grain

crackers as a creamy and low-sodium DASH Diet dip.

Nutritional Information (per serving): 80 calories, 3g protein, 6g carbohydrates, 5g fat, 1g saturated fat, 75mg sodium

131. COCONUT & DARK CHOCOLATE KEFIR PARFAIT

Cooking time: 10mins   **Yield:** 2

Ingredients

- 1 cup low-fat coconut kefir
- 1/4 cup dark chocolate chips
- 1/4 cup granola
- 1/4 cup fresh berries (blueberries, strawberries)
- 1/4 teaspoon salt

Instructions

- In serving glasses, layer low-fat coconut kefir, dark chocolate chips, granola, and fresh berries.
- Layers should be repeated until the glasses are full.
- Sprinkle a pinch of salt on top.
- Serve the Coconut & Dark Chocolate Kefir Parfait as a delightful and low-sodium DASH Diet dessert or breakfast.

Nutritional Information (per serving): 200 calories, 5g protein, 25g carbohydrates, 9g fat, 5g saturated fat, 50mg sodium

132.   BLUEBERRY BLING

Cooking time: 5 mins   **Yield:** 1

Ingredients

- 1 cup fresh blueberries
- 1 tablespoon chopped walnuts
- 1 tablespoon honey
- 1/4 teaspoon cinnamon
- 1/4 teaspoon salt

Instructions

- In a bowl, combine fresh blueberries, chopped walnuts, honey, cinnamon, and salt.
- Mix the items thoroughly by giving them a gentle toss.
- Serve the Blueberry Bling as a quick and low-sodium DASH Diet snack or dessert.

Nutritional Information (per serving): 120 calories, 2g protein, 20g carbohydrates, 5g fat, 0.5g saturated fat, 50mg sodium

133.   BAKED STUFFED APPLES

Cooking time: 40 mins   **Yield:** 4

Ingredients

- 4 medium-sized apples, cored
- 1/2 cup chopped nuts (walnuts or almonds)
- 1/4 cup dried cranberries
- 2 tablespoons honey
- 1 teaspoon cinnamon
- 1/4 teaspoon salt

Instructions

- Adjust the oven temperature to 375°F (190°C) and coat a baking dish with oil.
- In a bowl, mix chopped nuts, dried cranberries, honey, cinnamon, and salt.
- Stuff each cored apple with the nut mixture.
- Place the stuffed apples in the baking dish and bake for 25 minutes or until tender.
- Serve the Baked Stuffed Apples warm as a delectable and low-sodium DASH Diet dessert.

Nutritional Information (per serving): 150 calories, 2g protein, 30g carbohydrates, 5g fat, 0.5g saturated fat, 50mg sodium

134.   ALMOND RICE PUDDING

Cooking time: 2 hr 40 mins   **Yield:** 6

Ingredients

- 1 cup cooked brown rice
- 2 cups low-fat milk
- 1/4 cup honey
- 1/2 teaspoon almond extract
- 1/4 cup sliced almonds
- 1/4 teaspoon salt

Instructions

- In a saucepan, combine cooked brown rice, low-fat milk, honey, almond extract, and salt.
- Bring the mixture to a simmer and cook for 30 minutes, stirring occasionally.
- Remove from heat and stir in sliced almonds.
- Allow the almond rice pudding to cool, then refrigerate for at least 2 hours.
- Serve chilled as a creamy and low-sodium DASH Diet dessert.

Nutritional Information (per serving): 180 calories, 5g protein, 30g carbohydrates, 5g fat, 1g saturated fat, 80mg sodium

135. WHOOPIE PIES

Cooking time: 1 hr   **Yield:** 12

Ingredients

- 2 cups whole wheat flour
- 1/2 cup unsweetened cocoa powder
- Bake for 10 minutes or until the pies spring back when touched.
- Let the whoopie pies cool completely.
- For the filling, melt dark chocolate chips and stir in salt.
- Spread the chocolate filling on half of the whoopie pies and top with the remaining halves.

- 1 teaspoon baking soda
- 1/4 teaspoon salt
- 1 cup low-fat Greek yogurt
- 1/2 cup unsweetened applesauce
- 1/2 cup honey
- 1 teaspoon vanilla extract
- 1/4 cup dark chocolate chips (for filling)
- 1/4 teaspoon salt (for filling)

Instructions

- Adjust the oven temperature to 350°F (175°C) and place parchment paper on a baking pan.
- In a bowl, whisk together whole wheat flour, cocoa powder, baking soda, and salt.
- In another bowl, mix low-fat Greek yogurt, unsweetened applesauce, honey, and vanilla extract.
- Stirring until well blended, gradually add the dry ingredients to the wet ones.
- Drop tablespoon-sized portions of batter onto the prepared baking sheet.

- Serve the Whoopie Pies as a delightful and low-sodium DASH Diet dessert.

Nutritional Information (per serving): 150 calories, 3g protein, 30g carbohydrates, 3g fat, 1.5g saturated fat, 70mg sodium

136. HOMEMADE MOCHA S'MORES

Cooking time: 20 mins   **Yield:** 1

Ingredients

- 8 whole grain graham crackers
- 4 dark chocolate squares (70% cocoa)
- 4 marshmallows
- 1 shot of espresso
- 1/4 teaspoon cocoa powder
- Pinch of salt

Instructions

- Preheat the oven broiler.
- Place graham crackers on a baking sheet.
- Top each graham cracker with a square of dark chocolate and a marshmallow.
- Broil for 3-5 minutes or until marshmallows are golden.
- Meanwhile, prepare a shot of espresso.
- Once out of the oven, drizzle espresso over the s'mores.
- Sprinkle with cocoa powder and a pinch of salt.
- Serve the Homemade Mocha S'mores as a delightful and low-sodium DASH Diet dessert.

Nutritional Information (per serving): 120 calories, 2g protein, 20g carbohydrates, 5g fat, 2g saturated fat, 50mg sodium

137. COFFEE CAKE

Cooking time: 45 mins   **Yield:** 8

Ingredients

- One and a half cups whole wheat flour
- 1/2 cup rolled oats
- 1/2 cup unsweetened applesauce
- 1/4 cup honey
- 1/4 cup low-fat milk
- 2 tablespoons olive oil
- 1 teaspoon baking powder
- 1/2 teaspoon cinnamon
- 1/4 teaspoon salt

Instructions

- Turn the oven on to 350°F (175°C) and coat a baking dish with oil.
- Combine the whole wheat flour, rolled oats, honey, milk, applesauce, olive oil, baking powder, cinnamon, and salt in a bowl.
- Fill the baking dish with the batter.
- When a toothpick is inserted, bake for 30 minutes, or until it comes out clean.
- Allow the coffee cake to cool before slicing.
- Serve the Coffee Cake as a tasty and low-sodium DASH Diet breakfast or dessert.

Nutritional Information (per serving): 150 calories, 3g protein, 25g carbohydrates, 5g fat, 1g saturated fat, 60mg sodium

138. CHOCOLATE SHEET CAKE WITH PEANUT BUTTER FROSTING

Cooking time: 1 hr 45 mins   **Yield:** 12

Ingredients

- 1 1/2 cups whole wheat flour
- 1/2 cup unsweetened cocoa powder
- 1 teaspoon baking soda
- 1/2 teaspoon salt
- 1 cup low-fat milk
- 1/2 cup unsweetened applesauce
- 1/4 cup olive oil
- 1 cup coconut sugar
- 2 large eggs
- 1 teaspoon vanilla extract
- For Peanut Butter Frosting:
- 1/2 cup natural peanut butter
- 1/4 cup low-fat Greek yogurt
- 2 tablespoons honey
- Pinch of salt

Instructions

- Preheat the oven to 350°F (175°C) and grease a sheet cake pan.
- In a bowl, whisk together whole wheat flour, cocoa powder, baking soda, and salt.

- In another bowl, mix low-fat milk, applesauce, olive oil, coconut sugar, eggs, and vanilla extract.
- Stirring until well blended, gradually add the dry ingredients to the wet ones.
- Fill the sheet cake pan with the batter.
- When a toothpick is inserted, bake for 25 minutes, or until it comes out clean.
- Let the cake cool fully before applying the icing.
- For the peanut butter frosting, mix peanut butter, Greek yogurt, honey, and a pinch of salt until smooth.
- Spread the frosting over the chocolate sheet cake.
- Serve the Chocolate Sheet Cake with Peanut Butter Frosting as a decadent and low-sodium DASH Diet dessert.

Nutritional Information (per serving): 200 calories, 5g protein, 30g carbohydrates, 8g fat, 2g saturated fat, 70mg sodium

139. APPLE WALNUT CROSTATA

Cooking time: 45 mins   **Yield:** 8

Ingredients

- 1 store-bought whole wheat pie crust
- 4 cups thinly sliced apples (Granny Smith or Honeycrisp)
- 1/2 cup chopped walnuts
- 2 tablespoons honey

- 1 teaspoon cinnamon
- 1/4 teaspoon salt
- 1 tablespoon whole wheat flour (for dusting)

Instructions

- Before proceeding, preheat the oven to 375°F (190°C) and place parchment paper on a baking pan.
- Roll out the whole wheat pie crust on a floured surface.
- In a bowl, mix sliced apples, chopped walnuts, honey, cinnamon, and salt.
- Leaving a border around the apple mixture, place it in the middle of the pie shell.
- Fold the edges of the crust over the apple filling, creating a rustic shape.
- Dust the edges with whole wheat flour.
- Bake for 25 minutes or until the crust is golden and the apples are tender.
- Allow the crostata to cool slightly before slicing.
- Serve the Apple Walnut Crostata warm as a delightful and low-sodium DASH Diet dessert.

Nutritional Information (per serving): 180 calories, 3g protein, 25g carbohydrates, 8g fat, 1.5g saturated fat, 60mg sodium

140. CHOCOLATE PEPPERMINT CAKE

Cooking time: 1 hr 50 mins   **Yield:** 12

Ingredients

- One and a half cups whole wheat flour
- 1/2 cup unsweetened cocoa powder
- 1 1/2 teaspoons baking powder
- 1/2 teaspoon baking soda
- 1/4 teaspoon salt
- 1 cup low-fat milk
- 1/4 cup olive oil
- 1/2 cup honey
- 2 large eggs
- 1 teaspoon vanilla extract
- 1/2 teaspoon peppermint extract
- 1/4 cup dark chocolate chips (for topping)
- Crushed peppermint candies (for garnish)
- Pinch of salt

Instructions

- Grease a cake pan and set the the oven to 350°F (175°C).
- Mix the whole wheat flour, baking powder, baking soda, cocoa powder, and salt in a bowl.
- Combine low-fat milk, eggs, honey, olive oil, vanilla extract, peppermint essence, and a small amount of salt in a separate bowl.

- Stirring until well blended, gradually add the dry ingredients to the wet ones.
- Transfer the mixture into the ready-made cake pan.
- When a toothpick is inserted, bake for 30 minutes, or until it comes out clean.
- Let the cake cool fully before adding the topping.
- Melt dark chocolate chips and drizzle over the cake.
- Garnish with crushed peppermint candies.
- Serve the Chocolate Peppermint Cake as a decadent and low-sodium DASH Diet dessert.

Nutritional Information (per serving): 200 calories, 4g protein, 30g carbohydrates, 8g fat, 2g saturated fat, 70mg sodium

- Adjust the oven temperature to 375°F (190°C) and coat a baking dish with oil.
- In a bowl, mix chopped pecans, raisins, honey, cinnamon, and salt.
- Stuff each cored apple with the nut and fruit mixture.
- Place the stuffed apples in the baking dish.
- Add water to the dish's bottom.
- Bake for 25 minutes or until the apples are tender.
- Serve the Baked Apples warm as a comforting and low-sodium DASH Diet dessert.

Nutritional Information (per serving): 150 calories, 2g protein, 30g carbohydrates, 5g fat, 0.5g saturated fat, 50mg sodium

141.   BAKED APPLES

Cooking time: 40 mins   **Yield:** 4

Ingredients

- 4 large apples, cored
- 1/4 cup chopped pecans
- 2 tablespoons raisins
- 2 tablespoons honey
- 1 teaspoon cinnamon
- 1/4 teaspoon salt
- 1/2 cup water

Instructions

142.   BLUEBERRY PANNA COTTA

Cooking time: 4hrs 20mins   **Yield:** 4

Ingredients

- 1 cup low-fat milk
- 1 teaspoon unflavored gelatin
- 2 tablespoons honey
- 1 teaspoon vanilla extract
- 1 cup low-fat Greek yogurt
- 1/2 cup fresh blueberries
- Pinch of salt

Instructions

- In a saucepan, warm the milk without boiling.
- Sprinkle gelatin over the milk, allowing it to dissolve.
- Stir in honey and vanilla extract.
- Let the mixture cool slightly.
- In a bowl, whisk Greek yogurt until smooth.
- Gradually whisk in the milk mixture.
- Pour the panna cotta mixture into serving glasses.
- Chill for a minimum of four hours or until it is set.
- Top with fresh blueberries before serving.
- Sprinkle a pinch of salt for enhanced flavor.
- Serve the Blueberry Panna Cotta as a sophisticated and low-sodium DASH Diet dessert.

Nutritional Information (per serving): 120 calories, 6g protein, 15g carbohydrates, 4.5g fat, 2.5g saturated fat, 60mg sodium

143. FRESH ORANGE CREAM CHEESE FROSTING ON A CARROT CAKE

Cooking time: 1 hr 50 mins   **Yield:** 12

Ingredients

- 2 cups grated carrots
- 1/2 cup chopped walnuts
- 1/2 cup unsweetened applesauce
- 1/4 cup olive oil
- 2 large eggs
- 1/2 cup honey
- 1 teaspoon vanilla extract
- 1 1/2 cups whole wheat flour
- 1 teaspoon baking soda
- 1/2 teaspoon cinnamon
- For Fresh Orange Cream Cheese Frosting:
- 4 ounces low-fat cream cheese, softened
- 1/4 cup honey
- Zest of 1 orange
- Pinch of salt

Instructions

- Oil a cake pan and preheat the oven to 350°F (175°C).
- Grated carrots, chopped walnuts, applesauce, eggs, honey, and vanilla essence should all be combined in a bowl.
- Mix the cinnamon, baking soda, and whole wheat flour in a separate basin.
- Stirring until well blended, gradually add the dry ingredients to the wet ones.
- Transfer the mixture into the ready-made cake pan.
- When a toothpick is inserted, bake for 30 minutes, or until it comes out clean.
- Let the cake cool fully before applying the icing.

- For the orange cream cheese frosting, beat together cream cheese, honey, orange zest, and a pinch of salt until smooth.
- Spread the frosting over the carrot cake.
- Serve the Carrot Cake with Fresh Orange Cream Cheese Frosting as a delightful and low-sodium DASH Diet dessert.

Nutritional Information (per serving): 180 calories, 4g protein, 25g carbohydrates, 8g fat, 2g saturated fat, 70mg sodium

144. FRUIT PIZZA

Cooking time: 2 hrs 20 mins   **Yield:** 6

Ingredients

- 1 cup fresh raspberries
- 2 tablespoons honey
- 1 teaspoon lemon juice
- 1 cup low-fat Greek yogurt
- 1/4 cup unsweetened cocoa powder
- 2 tablespoons maple syrup
- Pinch of salt

Instructions

- In a blender, puree fresh raspberries, honey, and lemon juice until smooth.
- In a bowl, whisk together Greek yogurt, cocoa powder, maple syrup, and a pinch of salt.

- Gently fold the raspberry puree into the chocolate yogurt mixture.
- Spoon the mousse into individual cups.
- Chill for a minimum of two hours or until it is set.
- Garnish with additional raspberries before serving.
- Sprinkle a pinch of salt for balance.
- Serve the Chocolate Raspberry Mousse Cups as an indulgent and low-sodium DASH Diet dessert.

Nutritional Information (per serving): 110 calories, 5g protein, 15g carbohydrates, 3.5g fat, 2g saturated fat, 40mg sodium

145. CHOCO-NUT CAKE

Cooking time: 1 hr 50 mins   **Yield:** 12

Ingredients

- 1 1/2 cups whole wheat flour
- 1/2 cup unsweetened cocoa powder
- 1 1/2 teaspoons baking powder
- 1/2 teaspoon baking soda
- 1/4 cup olive oil
- 1/2 cup honey
- 2 large eggs
- 1 teaspoon vanilla extract
- 1/2 cup chopped walnuts
- 1/4 cup dark chocolate chips
- 1 cup low-fat milk
- Pinch of salt

Instructions

- Oil a cake pan and preheat the oven to 350°F (175°C).
- Mix the whole wheat flour, baking soda, baking powder, cocoa powder, and a small amount of salt in a basin.
- Combine the eggs, honey, vanilla essence, and olive oil in a separate bowl.
- Stirring until well blended, gradually add the dry ingredients to the wet ones.
- Add the dark chocolate chips and chopped walnuts and stir.
- Low-fat milk should be added to the batter gradually.
- Transfer the mixture into the ready-made cake pan.
- When a toothpick is inserted, bake for 30 minutes, or until it comes out clean.
- Before serving, let the cake cool fully.
- Sprinkle a pinch of salt over the top for enhanced flavor.
- Serve the Choco-Nut Cake as a rich and low-sodium DASH Diet dessert.

Nutritional Information (per serving): 180 calories, 4g protein, 25g carbohydrates, 8g fat, 2g saturated fat, 70mg sodium.

CHAPTER 9

BEVERAGES AND SMOOTHIES

146. BLACKBERRY ICED TEA WITH CINNAMON AND GINGER

Total Time: 2 hr 15 minutes   **Yield:** 4

Ingredients

- 4 cups water
- 4 black tea bags
- 1 cup fresh blackberries
- 1 teaspoon ground cinnamon
- 1 tablespoon fresh ginger, grated
- 2 tablespoons honey
- 1 tablespoon lemon juice
- Ice cubes
- Fresh blackberries and lemon slices for garnish
- Pinch of salt

Instructions

- Bring 4 cups of water to a boil and steep the black tea bags for 5 minutes.
- In a blender, combine fresh blackberries, ground cinnamon, grated ginger, honey, and lemon juice.
- Blend until smooth.
- Strain the blackberry mixture into the brewed tea, discarding solids.
- Let the tea cool until it reaches room temperature.
- Refrigerate for at least 2 hours.
- Serve the Blackberry Iced Tea over ice, garnished with fresh blackberries and lemon slices.
- Sprinkle a pinch of salt for balance.
- Enjoy the refreshing Blackberry Iced Tea as a hydrating and low-sodium DASH Diet beverage.

Nutritional Information (per serving): 30 calories, 0g protein, 8g carbohydrates, 0g fat, 0g saturated fat, 10mg sodium

147. BLUEBERRY LAVENDER LEMONADE

Total Time: 2 hr 10 minutes   **Yield:** 4

Ingredients

- 1 cup fresh blueberries
- 2 tablespoons dried lavender buds
- 1 cup hot water
- 1/2 cup honey
- 1 cup fresh lemon juice
- 4 cups cold water
- Ice cubes
- Fresh blueberries and lavender sprigs for garnish
- Pinch of salt

Instructions

- In a heatproof bowl, combine dried lavender buds and hot water, allowing it to steep for 5 minutes.
- Strain the lavender-infused water into a pitcher.
- In a blender, puree fresh blueberries and honey until smooth.
- Add the blueberry mixture to the pitcher with lavender water.
- Stir in fresh lemon juice and cold water.
- Refrigerate for at least 2 hours.
- Serve the Blueberry Lavender Lemonade over ice, garnished with fresh blueberries and lavender sprigs.
- Sprinkle a pinch of salt for enhanced flavor.
- Sip on this delightful Blueberry Lavender Lemonade as a soothing and low-sodium DASH Diet beverage.

Nutritional Information (per serving): 40 calories, 0g protein, 11g carbohydrates, 0g fat, 0g saturated fat, 10mg sodium

148. MANGO-GINGER SMOOTHIE

Total Time: 10 minutes   Yield: 2

Ingredients

1 cup frozen mango chunks

- 1 cup low-fat yogurt

- 1 tablespoon fresh ginger, grated
- 1 tablespoon honey
- 1/2 cup cold water
- Ice cubes
- Fresh mint leaves for garnish
- Pinch of salt

Instructions

- In a blender, combine frozen mango chunks, low-fat yogurt, grated ginger, honey, and cold water.
- Blend until smooth.
- Add ice cubes and blend again for a slushy consistency.
- Pour the Mango-Ginger Smoothie into glasses.
- Garnish with fresh mint leaves.
- Sprinkle a pinch of salt for balance.
- Enjoy the invigorating Mango-Ginger Smoothie as a nutrient-packed and low-sodium DASH Diet beverage.

Nutritional Information (per serving): 120 calories, 5g protein, 25g carbohydrates, 1.5g fat, 1g saturated fat, 60mg sodium

149. CHAMPAGNE FOOLER

Total Time: 5 minutes   Yield: 2

Ingredients

- 1 cup chilled champagne
- 1/2 cup cranberry juice (unsweetened)
- 1/4 cup sparkling water

- 1 tablespoon honey
- Fresh mint leaves for garnish
- Ice cubes
- Pinch of salt

Instructions

- In a pitcher, combine chilled champagne, cranberry juice, sparkling water, and honey.
- Stir until well mixed.
- Pour the Champagne Fooler into glasses over ice cubes.
- Garnish with fresh mint leaves.
- Sprinkle a pinch of salt for balance.
- Sip on this sophisticated Champagne Fooler as a light and low-sodium DASH Diet beverage.

Nutritional Information (per serving): 70 calories, 0g protein, 10g carbohydrates, 0g fat, 0g saturated fat, 10mg sodium

150.   CRANBERRY SPRITZER

Total Time: 5 minutes   **Yield:** 2

Ingredients

- 1 cup cranberry juice (unsweetened)
- 1/2 cup sparkling water
- 1 tablespoon fresh lime juice
- 1 tablespoon agave syrup
- Lime slices for garnish
- Ice cubes
- Pinch of salt

Instructions

- In a pitcher, combine cranberry juice, sparkling water, fresh lime juice, and agave syrup.
- Stir until well combined.
- Pour the Cranberry Spritzer into glasses over ice cubes.
- Garnish with lime slices.
- Sprinkle a pinch of salt for enhanced flavor.
- Enjoy the refreshing Cranberry Spritzer as a tangy and low-sodium DASH Diet beverage.

Nutritional Information (per serving): 50 calories, 0g protein, 12g carbohydrates, 0g fat, 0g saturated fat, 10mg sodium

151.   FRESH FRUIT SMOOTHIE

Total Time: 5 minutes   **Yield:** 2

Ingredients

- 1 cup mixed fresh fruits (such as berries, mango, and banana)
- 1/2 cup low-fat yogurt
- 1/2 cup cold water
- 1 tablespoon honey
- Ice cubes
- Fresh mint leaves for garnish
- Pinch of salt

Instructions

- In a blender, combine mixed fresh fruits, low-fat yogurt, cold water, and honey.
- Blend until smooth.
- Blend one more after adding the ice cubes for calming consistency.
- Pour the Fresh Fruit Smoothie into glasses.
- Garnish with fresh mint leaves.
- Sprinkle a pinch of salt for balance.
- Savor this nutritious Fresh Fruit Smoothie as a vibrant and low-sodium DASH Diet beverage.

Nutritional Information (per serving): 100 calories, 3g protein, 20g carbohydrates, 1g fat, 0.5g saturated fat, 60mg sodium

152.   GREEN SMOOTHIE

Total Time: 5 minutes   **Yield:** 2

Ingredients

- 2 cups fresh spinach leaves
- 1/2 cup cucumber, chopped
- 1/2 avocado, peeled and pitted
- 1 green apple, cored and chopped
- 1 tablespoon chia seeds
- 1 cup cold water
- Ice cubes
- Fresh mint leaves for garnish
- Pinch of salt

Instructions

- In a blender, combine fresh spinach leaves, chopped cucumber, avocado, green apple, chia seeds, and cold water.
- Blend until smooth.
- Blend one more after adding the ice cubes for calming consistency.
- Pour the Green Smoothie into glasses.
- Garnish with fresh mint leaves.
- Sprinkle a pinch of salt for balance.
- Enjoy this nutrient-packed Green Smoothie as a revitalizing and low-sodium DASH Diet beverage.

Nutritional Information (per serving): 120 calories, 4g protein, 15g carbohydrates, 7g fat, 1g saturated fat, 60mg sodium

153.   HURRICANE PUNCH

Total Time: 2 hr 10 minutes   **Yield:** 4

Ingredients

- 1 cup pineapple juice (unsweetened)
- 1/2 cup orange juice (unsweetened)
- 1/4 cup cranberry juice (unsweetened)
- 1 tablespoon fresh lime juice
- 1 tablespoon agave syrup
- 1 cup cold water
- Pineapple and orange slices for garnish
- Ice cubes
- Pinch of salt

Instructions

- In a pitcher, combine pineapple juice, orange juice, cranberry juice, fresh lime juice, agave syrup, and cold water.
- Stir until well mixed.
- Refrigerate for at least 2 hours.
- Serve the Hurricane Punch over ice, garnished with pineapple and orange slices.
- Sprinkle a pinch of salt for enhanced flavor.
- Sip on this tropical Hurricane Punch as a delightful and low-sodium DASH Diet beverage

Nutritional Information (per serving): 60 calories, 0g protein, 15g carbohydrates, 0g fat, 0g saturated fat, 10mg sodium

154. ICED LATTE

Total Time: 5 minutes   **Yield:** 2

Ingredients

- 1 cup strong brewed coffee, chilled
- 1/2 cup low-fat milk
- 1 tablespoon honey
- Ice cubes
- Pinch of salt

Instructions

- In a glass, combine strong brewed coffee, low-fat milk, and honey.
- Stir until honey is dissolved.

- Add ice cubes.
- Sprinkle a pinch of salt for balance.
- Enjoy the Iced Latte as a refreshing and low-sodium DASH Diet beverage.

Nutritional Information (per serving): 30 calories, 1g protein, 6g carbohydrates, 0g fat, 0g saturated fat, 30mg sodium

155. STRAWBERRY-BANANA PROTEIN SMOOTHIE

Total Time: 5 minutes   **Yield:** 2

Ingredients

- 1 cup fresh strawberries, hulled
- 1 ripe banana
- 1/2 cup low-fat Greek yogurt
- 1 scoop vanilla protein powder
- 1 tablespoon almond butter
- 1 cup cold water
- Ice cubes
- Pinch of salt

Instructions

- In a blender, combine fresh strawberries, ripe banana, low-fat Greek yogurt, vanilla protein powder, almond butter, and cold water.
- Blend until smooth.
- Blend one more after adding the ice cubes for calming consistency.
- Pour the Strawberry-Banana Protein Smoothie into glasses.

- Sprinkle a pinch of salt for balance.
- Enjoy this protein-packed smoothie as a satisfying and low-sodium DASH Diet beverage

Nutritional Information (per serving): 180 calories, 15g protein, 25g carbohydrates, 4g fat, 1g saturated fat, 90mg sodium

156. BERRY-ALMOND SMOOTHIE BOWL

Total Time: 5 minutes   **Yield:** 2

Ingredients

- 1 cup mixed berries (strawberries, blueberries, raspberries)
- 1 ripe banana
- 1/2 cup low-fat Greek yogurt
- 2 tablespoons almond butter
- 1 tablespoon chia seeds
- ¼ cup granola
- Fresh mint leaves for garnish
- Pinch of salt

Instructions

- In a blender, combine mixed berries, ripe banana, low-fat Greek yogurt, almond butter, and chia seeds.
- Blend until smooth.
- Pour the Berry-Almond Smoothie into bowls.
- Top with granola and fresh mint leaves.

- Sprinkle a pinch of salt for enhanced flavor.
- Indulge in this nutritious and low-sodium DASH Diet Smoothie Bowl.

Nutritional Information (per serving): 220 calories, 10g protein, 30g carbohydrates, 8g fat, 1g saturated fat, 80mg sodium

157. STRAWBERRY-CHOCOLATE SMOOTHIE

Total Time: 5 minutes   **Yield:** 2

Ingredients

- 1 cup fresh strawberries, hulled
- 1 ripe banana
- 1 tablespoon unsweetened cocoa powder
- 1 tablespoon chocolate protein powder
- 1 cup low-fat milk
- 1 tablespoon honey
- Ice cubes
- Pinch of salt

Instructions

- In a blender, combine fresh strawberries, ripe banana, unsweetened cocoa powder, chocolate protein powder, low-fat milk, and honey.
- Blend until smooth.

- Blend one more after adding the ice cubes for calming consistency.
- Pour the Strawberry-Chocolate Smoothie into glasses.
- Sprinkle a pinch of salt for balance.
- Delight in this decadent and low-sodium DASH Diet beverage.

Nutritional Information (per serving): 160 calories, 7g protein, 30g carbohydrates, 3g fat, 1g saturated fat, 70mg sodium

- Blend one more after adding the ice cubes for chilling consistency.
- Pour the Spinach-Avocado Smoothie into glasses.
- Sprinkle a pinch of salt for balance.
- Enjoy this nutrient-packed smoothie as a refreshing and low-sodium DASH Diet beverage.

Nutritional Information (per serving): 150 calories, 6g protein, 20g carbohydrates, 7g fat, 1g saturated fat, 70mg sodium

158. SPINACH-AVOCADO SMOOTHIE

Total Time: 5 minutes   **Yield:** 2

Ingredients

- 2 cups fresh spinach leaves
- 1/2 avocado, peeled and pitted
- 1 ripe banana
- 1/2 cup low-fat Greek yogurt
- 1 tablespoon chia seeds
- 1 cup cold water
- Ice cubes
- Pinch of salt

Instructions

- In a blender, combine fresh spinach leaves, avocado, ripe banana, low-fat Greek yogurt, chia seeds, and cold water.
- Blend until smooth.

159. MINTY-LIME ICED TEA

Total Time: 2 hr 10 minutes **Yield:** 4

Ingredients

- 4 cups cold water
- 4 green tea bags
- 1/4 cup fresh mint leaves
- 2 tablespoons fresh lime juice
- 2 tablespoons honey
- Lime slices and mint sprigs for garnish
- Ice cubes
- Pinch of salt

Instructions

- Heat two cups of water in a saucepan until it boils.
- Add green tea bags and fresh mint leaves. Steep for 5 minutes.
- Remove tea bags and mint leaves.

- Stir in fresh lime juice and honey.
- Pour the tea into a pitcher and add 2 cups of cold water.
- Refrigerate for at least 2 hours.
- Serve the Minty-Lime Iced Tea over ice, garnished with lime slices and mint sprigs.
- Sprinkle a pinch of salt for enhanced flavor.
- Sip on this cool and low-sodium DASH Diet beverage.

Nutritional Information (per serving): 20 calories, 0g protein, 5g carbohydrates, 0g fat, 0g saturated fat, 10mg sodium

160. STRAWBERRY BANANA MILKSHAKE

Total Time: 5 minutes   **Yield:** 2

Ingredients

- 1 cup fresh strawberries, hulled
- 1 ripe banana
- 1/2 cup low-fat milk
- 1/2 cup low-fat Greek yogurt
- 1 tablespoon honey
- 1/2 teaspoon vanilla extract
- Ice cubes
- Pinch of salt

Instructions

- In a blender, combine fresh strawberries, ripe banana, low-fat milk, low-fat Greek yogurt, honey, and vanilla extract.
- Blend until smooth.
- Add ice cubes and blend again for a frosty consistency.
- Pour the Strawberry Banana Milkshake into glasses.
- Sprinkle a pinch of salt for balance.
- Indulge in this creamy and low-sodium DASH Diet treat.

Nutritional Information (per serving): 140 calories, 5g protein, 30g carbohydrates, 1g fat, 0.5g saturated fat, 60mg sodium

CHAPTER 10

DIFFERENT EXERCISES TO COMBINE WITH THE DASH DIET RECIPES

There is more to starting a health journey than merely eating mindfully. This chapter explores the mutually beneficial relationship that exists between physical exercise and the DASH (Dietary Approaches to Stop Hypertension) diet. As we delve into a variety of activities designed to support your DASH lifestyle, you'll learn how the combination of wholesome recipes and intentional movement can enhance the advantages for your general health.

This chapter offers a carefully chosen collection of exercises that go well with your DASH diet journey, regardless of your level of experience or desire to start exercising regularly. Every workout has been carefully selected to improve muscular strength, cardiovascular health, and balance.

Are you prepared to strengthen your resolve to lead a healthier lifestyle? Together, we will begin on a fitness adventure that goes well with the healthy meals found in this cookbook. Now let's explore the main topic of the chapter, which is how exercise and the DASH diet work together to promote maximum health.

ADDING EXERCISES TO YOUR DIET: AN INTRODUCTION

Researchers at Duke University Medical Center found that adding exercise and weight loss to the nationally recommended DASH diet (Dietary Approaches to Stop Hypertension) decreased blood pressure at a rate comparable to those expected with medication use alone.

In a study published some time ago, blood pressure significantly improved (16 points) in DASH diet patients who engaged in aerobic exercise and were motivated to reduce weight. Patients who adhered to the diet alone saw an 11-point drop in blood pressure, whereas those in the control group who carried on with their regular lives saw an improvement of three points.

The study's lead author, a psychologist at Duke, said, "We were surprised by the extent of blood pressure drops in DASH diet participants who lost pounds and worked out, and we discovered that they also enhanced other critical cardiovascular biomarkers."

"Although not as much as those who also exercised and reduced weight, participants who only followed the DASH diet showed improvement."

National guidelines for blood pressure prevention and treatment include the DASH diet. Instead of emphasizing weight loss through meals consisting of fruits, vegetables, and low-fat dairy products, it places more emphasis on nutritional lifestyle modifications. Instead of fats, red meats, sweets, and sugar-filled beverages, whole grains, chicken, fish, and nuts are recommended.

This new study is the first to assess how the DASH diet affected individuals who chose and cooked their own meals yet, in certain circumstances, did not see weight loss. Since most previous research involved participants choosing their meals from a predetermined menu, Blumenthal claimed that this study is comparable to a "real world" experience.

The 'pre-hypertensive' and mildly hypertensive individuals included in the study represent a significant percent of our population," Blumenthal stated. "We may have the chance to stop heart attacks and strokes in the future if we can step in and make adjustments at this crucial point in the process.

Among the 144 participants were those who were fat or overweight, did not take medication, and had high blood pressure (diastolic: 85–99 and systolic: 130–159). They were divided into three groups at random: those who followed the DASH diet alone, those who followed it in addition to aerobic activity and small group discussions about weight loss strategies, and those who did not alter their exercise or food habits.

The exercise and weight management group shed an average of about 19 pounds after four months, whereas the other two groups either gained weight or lost very little. Apart from variations in blood pressure, the research team also noticed alterations in the composition and operation of the heart. Heart arterial stiffness and left ventricular thickness were reduced in DASH diet-following weight-loss and activity participants.

Blood pressure is a predictor of disease risk, Blumenthal noted that other biomarkers they looked at are the effects of high blood pressure exposure, which are significant independent predictors of cardiovascular morbidity and mortality. The DASH diet idea was presented to all participants by the research team following the four-month study period. They are keeping an eye on these people to see how much they adhere to the diet and how it affects blood pressure and other illness markers.

WORKOUTS FOR DIFFERENT FITNESS LEVELS

BEGINNER LEVEL

- **Cardiovascular Kickstart**
  - 10-minute brisk walking or light jogging
  - 5 minutes of jumping jacks
  - 10 minutes of cycling or stationary biking
- **Foundation Strength**
  - Bodyweight exercises: squats, lunges, push-ups (modified if needed)
  - 15 minutes of beginner-friendly yoga or stretching routine
  - Introduction to resistance bands for added challenge

INTERMEDIATE LEVEL

- **Elevated Cardio**
  - 20-minute run or brisk cycling
  - 10 minutes of high-intensity interval training (HIIT) like jumping rope or sprint intervals
- **Progressive Strength**
  - Bodyweight exercises with added resistance: squats, lunges, push-ups
  - 20 minutes of strength training with dumbbells or kettlebells
  - Introduction to more complex yoga poses for balance and flexibility
- **Cross-Training Fusion**
  - 30 minutes of swimming or water aerobics
  - 15 minutes of circuit training combining cardio and strength exercises

ADVANCED LEVEL

- **Intense Cardio Fusion**
  - 30-minute high-intensity run or cycling
  - 15 minutes of plyometric exercises (box jumps, burpees)
  - Incorporation of agility drills for enhanced cardiovascular challenge
- **Advanced Strength Challenge**
  - Weighted exercises: squats, deadlifts, bench press

- 20 minutes of advanced bodyweight exercises (handstand push-ups, pistol squats)
  - Introduction to advanced yoga flows for increased strength and flexibility
- **Endurance and Power**
  - 45 minutes of trail running or advanced cycling
  - 20 minutes of powerlifting-style training, focusing on explosive movements

TRAINING SCHEDULE TO PAIR WITH DASH DIET

WEEK 1-2: ESTABLISHING FOUNDATIONS

- **Monday:**
  - Morning: 15-minute brisk walk or light jog
  - Evening: Foundation strength workout (bodyweight exercises)
- **Wednesday:**
  - Morning: 20-minute cycling
  - Evening: Beginner-friendly yoga or stretching routine
- **Friday:**
  - Morning: 10-minute jumping jacks, 10-minute stationary biking
  - Evening: Resistance band workout

WEEK 3-4: BUILDING CARDIOVASCULAR ENDURANCE

- **Monday:**
  - Morning: 20-minute run
  - Evening: Progressive strength workout (bodyweight exercises with added resistance)
- **Wednesday:**
  - Morning: 15-minute sprint intervals
  - Evening: Introduction to complex yoga poses
- **Friday:**
  - Morning: 30-minute high-intensity cycling
  - Evening: Cross-training fusion (circuit combining cardio and strength exercises)

WEEK 5-6: ADVANCING TO HIGHER INTENSITY

- **Monday:**
  - o Morning: 30-minute high-intensity run
  - o Evening: Advanced strength challenge (weighted exercises)
- **Wednesday:**
  - o Morning: 15-minute plyometric exercises
  - o Evening: Advanced yoga flows for strength and flexibility
- **Friday:**
  - o Morning: 45-minute trail running
  - o Evening: Endurance and power workout (powerlifting-style training)

As we come to the end of this chapter, we have begun a journey that combines the transformative power of exercise with the DASH (Dietary Approaches to Stop Hypertension) diet's core principles. A route to holistic wellness is revealed by the interaction of intentional movement and mindful eating, where each aspect of wellness complements the other in a harmonious dance of health.

Thus range of exercises caters to a variety of fitness levels, from basic exercises for novices to more complex workouts requiring strength and endurance. The training schedule that is supplied serves as a roadmap, combining well with the DASH diet to produce a holistic approach to health. Keep in mind that your journey is distinct. Pay attention to your body, acknowledge your progress, and accept the changing relationship between food and exercise. I hope this chapter has provided you with motivation and useful ideas to promote long-lasting health.

Let this be more than just a chapter in your life; let it be a first step toward a way of living that embraces the nourishing DASH diet and the energizing power of intentional exercise. Cheers to living a life that is vibrant, in balance, and seamlessly integrates exercise and the DASH diet.

I WISH YOU HAPPY, HEALTHY EATING WITH NO REGRETS!

.

CONCLUSION

In the journey through the "Dash Diet Cookbook for Beginners 2024," we've explored not just a collection of recipes but a holistic approach to embracing a heart-healthy lifestyle. From the inception of the book, where we delved into the compelling narrative of a Dietitian's patient and their transformative journey with the DASH Diet, to the comprehensive overview of the DASH Diet itself, every page has been a step toward a healthier, more balanced life.

RECAP OF DASH DIET PRINCIPLES

In wrapping up our culinary odyssey through the "Dash Diet Cookbook for Beginners 2024," it's crucial to recap the foundational principles that underpin the DASH Diet. This lifestyle isn't just about the recipes; it's about embracing a holistic approach to health that extends beyond the plate. Let's revisit the key principles that make the DASH Diet a powerful and sustainable guide to wellness:

1. Sodium Sensibility: At the heart of the DASH Diet lies a conscious effort to reduce sodium intake. By curbing our salt consumption, we actively contribute to lower blood pressure and overall cardiovascular health. The recipes in this book have been crafted with this principle in mind, ensuring that flavor is not sacrificed, even as we prioritize heart health.

2. Nutrient-Rich Choices: The DASH Diet champions the consumption of nutrient-dense foods. We've celebrated a spectrum of fresh fruits, vibrant vegetables, whole grains, lean proteins, and low-fat dairy throughout the book. These choices provide essential vitamins, minerals, and antioxidants, nourishing our bodies at the cellular level.

3. Balanced Macronutrients: The DASH Diet doesn't advocate extreme measures but encourages a balanced approach to macronutrients. With a focus on incorporating the right proportions of carbohydrates, proteins, and healthy fats, each recipe becomes a harmonious ensemble that supports overall well-being.

4. Portion Moderation: Size matters, and the DASH Diet emphasizes mindful portion control. By understanding serving sizes and being mindful of our eating habits, we prevent overindulgence and maintain a healthy weight. The recipes provided are designed with moderation in mind, promoting a sustainable and enjoyable relationship with food.

5. Exercise Integration: Beyond the kitchen, the DASH Diet extends its influence into our daily physical activity. The incorporation of exercise into this culinary journey is a reminder that a comprehensive approach to health involves not only what we eat but also how we move. Together, these elements form a potent recipe for a resilient heart and an active lifestyle.

ENCOURAGEMENT FOR CONTINUED SUCCESS

Now that I am about to wrap up this amazing guide, it's also essential to instill a sense of encouragement for the road that lies ahead. Embarking on a lifestyle change, particularly one as transformative as the DASH Diet, is an ongoing commitment to your well-being. Here's a heartfelt encouragement to foster your continued success:

1. Celebrate Progress, Not Perfection: Every step you take toward adopting the DASH Diet is a triumph. Embrace the journey with kindness and celebrate your progress, recognizing that sustainable change is a gradual process. Remember, each meal prepared with health in mind is a step toward a more vibrant and resilient you.

2. Embrace Flexibility: Life is dynamic, and so are our circumstances. The DASH Diet is flexible, allowing for adaptation to various preferences and lifestyles. If you encounter challenges or deviations, view them as opportunities to learn and adjust. The key is to find a rhythm that resonates with your unique needs.

3. Build a Support System: Change is often more enjoyable when shared. Consider involving friends, family, or loved ones in your DASH Diet journey. Share recipes, embark on cooking adventures together, or engage in physical activities as a group. A supportive community can provide motivation, inspiration, and a sense of camaraderie.

4. Listen to Your Body: Your body communicates its needs, and tuning in to these signals is crucial. Pay attention to hunger and fullness cues, adapt recipes to suit your taste preferences, and be attuned to how different foods make you feel. The DASH Diet is a personalized experience, and listening to your body is a powerful compass for sustained success.

5. Set Realistic Goals: Establishing achievable goals is fundamental to long-term success. Whether it's committing to more plant-based meals, incorporating new recipes weekly, or gradually increasing your physical activity, setting realistic goals ensures a sense of accomplishment and motivates you to persist on this transformative path.

6. Prioritize Self-Care: The DASH Diet extends beyond food and exercise; it's about holistic well-being. Prioritize self-care, encompassing adequate sleep, stress management, and mindfulness. A well-nurtured mind and body create a resilient foundation for embracing the DASH lifestyle with joy and fulfillment.

As we conclude this culinary and lifestyle journey, it's crucial to recognize that the DASH Diet is not a short-term fix but a sustainable way of life. The recipes provided aren't just ingredients thrown together; they are building blocks for a healthier, happier future. Every meal prepared with the principles of the DASH Diet becomes a contribution to overall wellness.

Let this book serve as a guide, a companion on your quest for health. Whether you're a seasoned health enthusiast or a newcomer to the world of nutrition, the DASH Diet Cookbook for Beginners 2024 invites you to embark on a flavorful journey toward a heart-healthy lifestyle. May your kitchen become a sanctuary for nourishment, and may each bite be a step toward a brighter, healthier tomorrow.

Wishing you strength, joy, and continued success on your renal wellness adventure.

WARM REGARDS,

JUANITA SCOTT.

AUTHOR, FATTY LIVER DIET COOKBOOK FOR SENIORS AND BEGINNERS

COOKING CONVERSION CHARTS

MEASUREMENTS

CUPS	OUNCES	MILLILITERS	TABLESPOONS
8 cups	64 oz	1895 mil	128
6 cups	48 oz	1420 mil	96
5 cups	40 oz	1120 mil	80
4 cups	32 oz	960 mil	64
2 cup	16 oz	480 mil	32
1 cup	8 oz	240 mil	16
¾ cup	6 oz	177 mil	12
⅔ cup	5 oz	158 mil	11
½ cup	4 oz	118 mil	8
⅜ cup	3 oz	90 mil	6
⅓ cup	2.5 oz	79 mil	5.5
¼ cup	2 oz	59 mil	4
⅛ cup	1 oz	30 mil	3
1/16 cup	½ oz	15 mil	1

TEMPERATURE

FAHRENHEIT	CELCIUS
100 °F	37 °C
150 °F	65 °C
200 °F	93 °C
250 °F	121 °C
300 °F	150 °C
325 °F	160 °C
350 °F	180 °C
375 °F	190 °C
400 °F	200 °C
425 °F	220 °C
450 °F	230 °C
500 °F	260 °C
525 °F	274 °C
550 °F	288 °C

WEIGHT

IMPERIAL	METRIC
½ oz	15 g
1 oz	29 g
2 oz	57 g
3 oz	85 g
4 oz	113 g
5 oz	141 g
6 oz	170 g
8 oz	227 g
10 oz	283 g
12 oz	340 g
13 oz	369 g
14 oz	397 g
15 oz	425 g
1 lb	453 g

A DEEP REQUEST

Dearest Reader,

I hope you've had the chance to dive into "The Dash Diet Cookbook for Beginners 2024." Your opinion matters greatly, and I would be honored to hear your thoughts. Your honest reviews play a crucial role in helping others discover the benefits of this comprehensive guide.

Whether you've tried the recipes, followed the meal plan, or simply enjoyed the insights shared, your feedback is invaluable. Please take a moment to share your thoughts on platforms like Amazon, Goodreads, or any other platform where you obtained your copy.

Your reviews not only guide future readers but also contribute to the ongoing conversation about kidney health. Thank you for being a part of this journey, and I look forward to hearing from you.

RECOMMENDED READING

Dearest Esteemed Reader,

I trust you're enjoying "The Dash Diet Cookbook for Beginners 2024" and finding it beneficial on your health journey. If you've been inspired by my approach to wellness, I'd like to introduce you to two more valuable resources in my collection — "Fatty Liver for Seniors and Beginners & The Renal Diet Cookbook For Beginners 2024."

These insightful guides are tailored to support you and your family in navigating the complexities of fatty liver, and the renal disease concerns, offering practical advice and a range of accessible strategies for seniors and beginners alike.

Explore more from my authorship by visiting my author page, where you'll discover a wealth of information designed to empower you on your path to better health. To visit my author page, all you need to do is scan the QR code below. The QR code will take you straight to my author page.

SCAN HERE!

Thank you for your continued support and trust in my commitment to providing comprehensive health resources.

Best regards,

Juanita Scott.

My Complete Dash Diet 30-Day Meal Plan

Day	Breakfast	Lunch	Dinner	Snacks/ Side Dish	Dessert	Beverag/ Smoothie
1	Sweet Potato Hash Browns	Baked Salmon with Roasted Vegetables	Baked Cod with Mediterranean Herbs	Cucumber and Tomato Salad	Yogurt with Fresh Strawberries and Honey	Blackberry Iced Tea with Cinnamon and Ginger
2	Quinoa Fruit Salad	Greek-Style Quinoa Salad	Baked Eggplant Parmesan	Greek Salad Skewers	Light Pumpkin Pie	Blueberry Lavender Lemonade
3	Cottage Cheese with Fruits	Vegetable Stir-Fry with Brown Rice	Mediterranean Couscous Salad	Kale Chips	Tahini and Almond Cookies	Mango-Ginger Smoothie
4	Yogurt with Granola and Fruit	Lemon Garlic Chicken with Asparagus	Lemon Garlic Chicken with Asparagus	Sliced Apple with Almond Butter	Oatmeal Walnut Chocolate Chip Cookies	Champagne Fooler
5	Quinoa Breakfast Porridge with Almond Butter	Lemon Herb Quinoa with Grilled Chicken	Honey Mustard Glazed Salmon	Cauliflower Popcorn	Pear-Cranberry Pie with Oatmeal Streusel	Cranberry Spritzer
6	Banana and Spinach Smoothies	Baked Chicken and Vegetable Foil Packets	Lemon Herb Quinoa with Grilled Chicken	Avocado and Salsa Dip	Milk Chocolate Pudding	Fresh Fruit Smoothie
7	Berry and Spinach Salad	Turkey and Vegetable Chili	Chickpea and Spinach Stew	Spinach and Tomato Frittata	Light and Easy Pear-Strawberry Trifle	Green Smoothie

8	Banana Walnut Muffins	Quinoa and Spinach Stuffed Peppers	Mexican Quinoa Skillet	Crispy Shrimp	Guilt-Free Banana Berry Ice Cream	Hurricane Punch
9	Veggie Frittata with Herbs	Ratatouille with Whole Wheat Couscous	Caprese Stuffed Chicken Breast	Apple Snack	Fabulous Fig Bars	Iced Latte
10	Homemade Muesli	Grilled Salmon with Lemon Dill Dressing	Ratatouille with Whole Wheat Couscous	Potato Crisp	California Skinny Dips	Strawberry-Banana Protein Smoothie
11	Tofu Scramble	Zucchini Noodles with Pesto	Italian Herb Grilled Pork Chops	Lentil Medley	Coconut & Dark Chocolate Kefir Parfait	Berry-Almond Smoothie Bowl
12	Blueberry and Almond Overnight Oats	Mediterranean Quinoa Salad	Spicy Shrimp Stir-Fry with Brown Rice	Spicy Almonds	Blueberry Bling	Strawberry-Chocolate Smoothie
13	Oatmeal with Mixed Berries	Caprese Sandwich with Pesto	Spice-Seared Salmon with Greek-Style Green Beans	Lentil Medley	Baked Stuffed Apples	Spinach-Avocado Smoothie
14	Tomatoes and Basil Omelets	Pumpkin Soup	One-Pan Chicken & Asparagus Bake	Spicy Almonds	Almond Rice Pudding	Minty-Lime Iced Tea
15	Veggie and Hummus Wrap	Bean Chili	Chickpea Pasta with Mushrooms & Kale	Lentil Medley	Whoopie Pies	Strawberry Banana Milkshake

16	Chicken Egg Wrap	Cauliflower Pizza	Lentil Stew with Salsa	Crispy Shrimp	Homemade Mocha S'mores	Strawberry Chocolate Smoothie
17	Sauteed Mushrooms with Egg	Baked Macaroni	Spice-Seared Salmon with Greek-Style Green Beans	Apple Snack	Coffee Cake	Berry-Almond Smoothie Bowl
18	Bullet Coffee	Brown Rice and Arugula Bowl	Roasted Salmon with Smoky Chickpeas & Greens	Apple Snack	Chocolate Sheet Cake with Peanut Butter Frosting	Minty-Lime Iced Tea
19	Apple Oats	Chicken Rice	Beef & Bean Sloppy Joes	Lentil Medley	Apple Walnut Crostata	Fresh Fruit Smoothie
20	Cheese Panini	Vegetarian Pita Meal	Sheet-Pan Chili-Lime Salmon with Potatoes & Peppers	Spicy Almonds	Chocolate Peppermint Cake	Mango-Ginger Smoothie
21	Quark Sandwich	Flat Bread Pizza	Sweet Potato Wedges and Brussels Sprouts with Maple-Roasted Chicken Thighs	Lentil Medley	Baked Apples	Strawberry-Banana Protein Smoothie
22	Broccoli Cheese Egg Muffins	Prawn Stew	One-Pan Chicken & Asparagus	Potato Crisp	Blueberry Panna Cott	Blackberry Iced Tea with Cinnamon and Ginger

23	Hard-Boiled Eggs	Greek Chicken Salad	Sheet-Pan Chili-Lime Salmon with Potatoes & Peppers	Lentil Medley	Fresh Orange Cream Cheese Frosting on a Carrot Cake	Blueberry Lavender Lemonade
24	Baked Avocado Eggs	Turkey and Vegetable Stir-Fry	Walnut-Rosemary Crusted Salmon	Spicy Almonds	Fruit Pizza	Mango-Ginger Smoothie
25	Peach Pancakes	Chicken and Vegetable Kabobs	One-Pot Garlicky Shrimp & Spinach	Apple Snack	Choco-Nut Cake	Cranberry Spritzer
26	Sweet Potato Hash Browns	Baked Cod with Lemon Pepper Sauce	Roasted Salmon	Kale Chips	Baked Stuffed Apples	Fresh Fruit Smoothie
27	Quinoa Fruit Salad	Oven Baked Tilapia	Crunchy Baked Fish	Cucumber and Tomato Salad	Almond Rice Pudding	Mango-Ginger Smoothie
28	Cottage Cheese with Fruits	Fish Tacos	Baked Lemon Salmon	Spinach and Tomato Frittata	Chocolate Sheet Cake with Peanut Butter Frosting	Blueberry Lavender Lemonade
29	Yogurt with Granola and fruits	Tuna Broccoli Pasta	Cajun Shrimp	Crispy Shrimp	Apple Walnut Crostata	Blackberry Iced Tea with Cinnamon and Ginge

30	Quinoa Breakfast Porridge with Almond Butter	Spicy Shrimp Stir Fry with Brown Rice	Baked Cod with Mediterranean Herbs	Avocado and Salsa Dip	Chocolate Peppermint Cake	Blueberry Lavender Lemonade

www.ingramcontent.com/pod-product-compliance
Lightning Source LLC
LaVergne TN
LVHW081128130425
808531LV00015B/1586